# The Paradox of Sleep

# The Paradox of Sleep
## The Story of Dreaming

Michel Jouvet
Translated by Laurence Garey

A Bradford Book
The MIT Press
Cambridge, Massachusetts
London, England

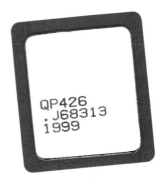
© 1999 Massachusetts Institute of Technology

This work originally appeared in French under the title *Le Sommeil et le Rêve*.

© 1993 Odile Jacob

Published with the help of the French Ministry of Culture—CNL.

This book was set in Sabon by Asco Typesetters, Hong Kong and was printed and bound in the United States of America.

Library of Congress Cataloging-in-Publication Data

Jouvet, Michel.
  [Sommeil et le rêve. English]
  The paradox of sleep : the story of dreaming / by Michel Jouvet ; translated by Laurence Garey.
     p.   cm.
  "A Bradford book."
  Includes bibliographical references and index.
  ISBN 0-262-10080-0 (alk. paper)
  1. Dreams. 2. Sleep. I. Title.
QP426.J68313   1999
612.8′21—dc21                                                  98-50198
                                                                    CIP

# Contents

# Translator's Introduction

A proud native of the Franche-Comté of France, where he fought in the "maquis" during the Second World War, Michel Jouvet is a member of the French Academy of Sciences and holds the Gold Medal of the CNRS (Centre National de la Recherche Scientifique). He is Emeritus Professor of Experimental Medicine at the University of Lyon, and was director of the CNRS Unit for the Neurobiology of Vigilance and of the INSERM Unit for Molecular Oneirology.

He spent a year in the laboratory of Horace Magoun in California in 1955, where exciting new discoveries were being made concerning an area in the brain that controls arousal and wakefulness (the reticular formation). His work with Magoun inspired him to develop refined electrophysiological techniques to investigate states of vigilance and learning in the brain when he returned to France. It was while working on that project in Lyon in 1958 that he made a fortuitous discovery that he describes in chapter 1, a discovery that changed his research goal, and his whole life. It led to his description in 1959 of *paradoxical sleep*, when the individual is neither asleep nor awake, but under the influence of a "new" third state of the brain. His work came soon after the discovery of rapid eye movement (REM) sleep by the group of neurophysiologists in

Chicago comprising Nathaniel Kleitman, William Dement, and Eugene Aserinsky, with whom he maintained close professional and amicable contacts.

Since then he has devoted himself to research on sleep and dreaming in his laboratories in Lyon. Although recently retired, he continues to work and to travel the world in pursuit of his goal of understanding how and why we dream. The team of students and disciples that he has formed over the years continues his everyday work and is delving into new realms.

The question of the relationship between REM sleep in man, paradoxical sleep in other animals, and dreaming in all, has remained a vexed one. Michel Jouvet has developed a number of theories about the *function* of dreaming rather than merely its *mechanism* ("why" as opposed to "how"). The most controversial of these theories is that dreaming may be an essential part of the maintenance of our individuality at the genetic level.

I well remember his visits in the 1980s to the Institute of Anatomy at the University of Lausanne, not far from Lyon, where I was working at the time, when he gave us some highly animated seminars on his discoveries in the field of dreaming. I also recall discussions with various members of our institute about the adjective "onirique," and whether the English "oneiric" was really acceptable!

So I was very happy when Michael Rutter of The MIT Press asked me to translate *Le Sommeil et le Rêve* and especially when Michel Jouvet encouraged me to take on the task. I am grateful for the support that both Michael and Michel have given me during the translation.

*Le Sommeil et le Rêve* was originally written in part as a series of articles, and I have taken the opportunity to try to smooth them into an integrated text. I have taken certain liberties in rearranging the contents of the chapters which will, I hope, make the new text accessible to a wide audience, whether the young researcher that Michel Jouvet declares the book to be aimed at in his preface, or interested nonphysiologists! If in doing so any of the original information or ideas have been lost I must accept full responsibility. However, we have taken the opportunity to bring the story right up to date.

Chapter 1 takes us straight into the labyrinth of sleep, setting out to state the philosophy behind Michel Jouvet's work, and why he became addicted to it. It also describes the discovery of paradoxical sleep. He sets this event in the context of contemporary and earlier research, and goes on to sketch the events that were to follow rapidly in his, and other, research laboratories. We also derive glimpses of the excitement of that time and the people and lands that became a part of Jouvet's life as he sought ever wider solutions to the enigma of sleeping and dreaming at the physiological, anatomical, biochemical and even genetic levels.

In chapter 2, we examine the solid scientific evidence for the mechanisms of sleeping and dreaming. In addition to the hard laboratory science, we touch on the metaphysical, the philosophical, and the psychological. Then in chapter 3 we are carried away into the realms of dream memories: what we recall of our dreams. We learn how correlation between dream recall and physiological observation of the brain's activity has enabled us to begin to understand when, and perhaps why, dreaming takes place. A number of fascinating anecdotes from dreamland provide a compelling background to what is, in fact, very sophisticated science.

In chapter 4, Jouvet introduces us to another of the achievements of his research team, the revelation of how an animal might behave if it were able to live out its dreams, instead of being in a state of almost complete muscular paralysis, as is the case during our normal dreaming. We also learn of a strange human equivalent of this *oneiric behavior.*

Chapter 5 touches on the relationships of sleep with the mind and consciousness. We reenter a world between physiology and a modern form of metaphysics. It leads smoothly to chapter 6 which attempts to delve into the problem of *why* we dream. Why do we spend time several times a day in a state of semiparalysis, exposed to potential danger, performing this necessary but mysterious function that is dreaming? Freud had his ideas on the subject, artificial intelligence experts have theirs, and Jouvet has his. Indeed, in chapter 7 he gives a detailed insight into his theory that we need regular, periodic dreaming to preserve our individuality, and that dreaming is a time for essential genetic reprogramming within our brain. This is a controversial, but fascinating debate.

Finally, chapter 8 consists of the reflections of a senior scientist about where all this has taken him and the scientific world around him.

In searching for a title for the English version, an alternative to "Sleep and Dreams" seemed desirable. I thought of Hamlet's premonition of sleep tormented by dreams, but Michael Rutter thought it just too obvious, and suggested the present title, which I find excellent. However, when I went back to the Bard's text, I thought it rather fitting, and hope I can be excused for reproducing it here:

*... by a sleep to say we end*
*The heart-ache and the thousand natural shocks*
*That flesh is heir to,—'tis a consummation*
*Devoutly to be wish'd. To die,—to sleep;—*
*To sleep! perchance to dream:—ay, there's the rub:*
*For in that sleep of death what dreams may come ...*

—William Shakespeare, *Hamlet*, Act III, Scene I

Laurence Garey, London, July 1998

# Preface to the French Edition

Many aspects of the objective study of dreaming still belong to the eighteenth century, when magic was invoked to explain the mysteries of reproduction, and the dialogue of the soul with animal spirits to explain dreams. The fact that we are so ignorant about the function of the brain should attract the most inquisitive and boldest scientists to Physiology, the Queen of Sciences. I wrote this book thinking of them.

"In the Labyrinth of Sleep" is a monologue which traces the life of a handful of neurobiologists. We see their adventures and their sometimes colorful travels, but also their hesitations. We see the numerous and inevitable technical and ideological obstacles that have marked research into the mechanisms and functions of sleeping and dreaming over forty years.

"The Natural History of Dreaming" is an open window on a research laboratory. I hope this simple but comprehensive account of the study of the science of dreams will stimulate a vocation in some researchers.

"Dream Memories" is dedicated to a nonanalytical approach to recalled memories of dreams. How long does it take for a phenomenon perceived during one's waking life to become incorporated in a dream? Readers who often travel to exotic lands, and who remember their dreams, must have noticed how strange it is to dream of one's home or workplace while in Amazonia or Nepal. Is there a dissociation between activity in the right and left cerebral hemispheres during dreams? How might we demonstrate it, using only dream recall? Analysis of the relationship between messages heard or seen in some dreams may be a starting point.

"Oneiric Behavior." The discovery of this phenomenon in the cat demonstrates that the frontiers between waking and dreaming can sometimes be difficult to define. What does a cat dream about? Recent discoveries on oneiric behavior in man, and on "lucid" dreams confirm that paradoxical sleep is indeed the objective reflection of dreaming.

"Sleep, the Other Side of the Spirit" attempts to answer the subtle question of a theologian during a conference in the Vatican. How can a neurobiologist talk of the spirit in the 1990s?

"The Functions of Dreaming" summarizes Freud's theory about both the "how" and the "why" of dreams. His theory is contrasted with modern data from the neurobiological study of dreaming. There is then a brief review of recent neurobiological theories about the functions of dreams.

"Is Paradoxical Sleep the Guardian of Psychological Individuality?" is intended for those who still believe that dreams, like the mind, are continuous throughout sleeping. It examines the latest developments of a theory of iterative programming of psychological individuation.

The book ends with an analysis of the evolution of the neurobiology of sleeping and dreaming since 1960 in the areas that will become familiar to the reader through the earlier chapters. The exponential development of the neurosciences over these years has helped overthrow certain theories or "paradigms." However, our ever preciser knowledge of the mechanisms, the "how" of dreams, has not yet enabled us to resolve the problem of "why." This is probably because here we have the greatest enigma that the dreaming brain offers to the waking brain.

# The Paradox of Sleep

# 1

# In the Labyrinth of Sleep

I do not believe that you need coherent behavior in science. Nor do I believe that you can "administer" research. If there was ever a field where there must be a maximum of freedom, it is science. To "administer" it would mean accepting a set of dogmas, a set of "facts." But by definition, the more you establish "facts," and the more publicity they get, the more chance there is they will block new lines of research.

On the other hand, I believe that the researcher has divine guidance. That is why I always rely on luck. Much of our work in the 1950s involved the then revolutionary technique of recording brain activity through tiny microelectrodes inserted in the living brain. One day in 1958, François Michel and I were studying the mechanism of learning in cats, and while placing a microelectrode in the brain of one, we were lucky.[85] Our experiment did not add much to our knowledge of learning, but it set us on a new path.

Some years earlier, the Chicago school of Nathaniel Kleitman, Eugene Aserinsky, and William Dement had discovered that during sleep there existed a period marked by rapid eye

Originally published as a conversation with Claire Parnet and Antoine Dulaure in the May 1990 issue of *L'Autre Journal*.

movements ("REM sleep") that was accompanied by dreams. They believed that REM sleep was a light stage of sleep ("emergent stage 1") analogous to the "descending stage 1" that occurred at the onset of sleep. Our finding, in the cat, led to an entirely different interpretation. It led, two or three years later, to our already knowing most of what we know now about the mysterious dream state that we named *paradoxical sleep*, and which will be the subject of this book. I used this expression, and still use it, to describe what we realized to be a *third* state of brain activity (in addition to sleeping and waking). It is a state of very deep sleep but, paradoxically, with some specific motor events, such as rapid movements of the eyes. However, compared with those first momentous discoveries, we have made only slow progress in the last forty years. What is more, the polemic it has created is still rife.

I worked for years on the question of energy related to sleep. From Monday morning to Friday night, without a break, we recorded from animals in conditions that allowed us to modify their body temperature without interference from their thermo-regulation systems. It is an art to reduce an animal's temperature very gradually. It is like piloting a million-ton tanker into port with a two-horsepower motor. You have to unconsciously weigh a host of factors: the weather outside, the thickness of the animal's coat, and so on. I have had so much trouble with all this that at least I now know the mistakes not to make. It is like the blacksmith's craft: you cannot describe it in words, either spoken or written. I still spend nights at the laboratory, sleeping when I can. I don't mind. Nights here are perfect: I can think, listen to the radio ...

Of course I should prefer to work in vitro, in brain tissue isolated from the animal itself, a sort of tissue culture. First, because it is much quicker, and also because it is fashionable!

Perhaps we could imagine sleep in vitro in ten years' time, when we know more about the energy involved in the process. But dreams in vitro? I cannot imagine that, although things we cannot conceive today might just happen! But I do not believe the present generation will live to see it. We shall have to continue with animals, or stop.

There are many examples in the history of science where whole realms of knowledge remained frozen for ten or twenty years, and then took off again. Take the case of dreaming. The first person to really try to relate it to sleep and look at its time course was Alfred Maury, who was a professor at the Collège de France in the late nineteenth century. The popular theory at the time was that the spirit, being immaterial, was constantly in motion, while the body underwent the "periodical death" of sleep. Alfred Maury managed to dispel this idea. He replaced it with his view of the dream as an episodic event *intermediate between sleep and wakefulness*. His concept has deeply influenced researchers who have studied the problem since.

We had to wait until the Second World War—for war always advances research!—to have access to instruments able to measure in microvolts in order to record the electrical activity of the brain during sleep.

In 1949 Giuseppe Moruzzi and Horace Magoun[112] discovered the *reticular formation*, part of the brain responsible for *arousal*, the term coined at the time to describe the state of alertness or waking (figure 1). For us this was a remarkable event. It looked as if there could be a simple explanation for sleep somewhere in the reticular formation. I shall come back to it in chapter 2.

To return to the findings of the Chicago school, in 1953 Eugene Aserinsky, a pupil of Nathaniel Kleitman, using a technique of placing electrodes on the outside of the scalp and face,

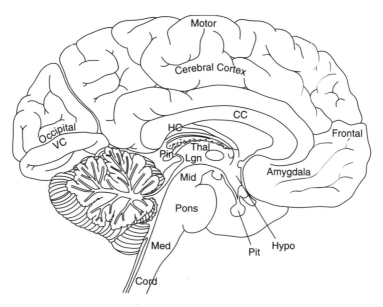

**Figure 1**
Diagram of the human brain seen from the inside surface (medial view). The front of the brain (anterior) is to the right. Various regions and structures of relevance to sleeping and dreaming are indicated to help understand their relationships from the text. Overlying most of the *cerebral hemisphere* is the *cerebral cortex*. Posteriorly is the cortex of the *occipital lobe* (*visual cortex*, VC). Anteriorly is the *frontal cortex*. The *motor cortex* is also marked. Deep to the medial part of the temporal cortex is the *amygdala*. The *corpus callosum* (CC) joins the left and right hemispheres. The *hippocampus* (HC) is just seen below the corpus callosum. The *lateral geniculate nucleus* (Lgn) of the *thalamus* (Thal), and the *hypothalamus* (Hypo) are visible. The latter contains several structures of interest to sleep research, including the *arcuate* and *preoptic* nuclei. The *pituitary gland* (Pit) "hangs" beneath the hypothalamus. The *pineal gland* (Pin) protrudes rearward behind the thalamus. The brainstem is composed of the *midbrain* (Mid), *pons*, and *medulla* (Med) and contains the *reticular formation* and many of the nuclei responsible for arousal and sleep, as described in the text.

observed periodic episodes of fast eye movements in sleeping infants. He called this phenomenon *rapid eye movement sleep* (usually shortened to *REM sleep*). His hypothesis was that it might correspond to periods of dreaming. But the subject's electroencephalogram (his "brain waves" or EEG) was like that of someone just falling to sleep. Maury's ideas were still in vogue, so Aserinsky and his colleagues concluded that dreaming was simply the *return of light sleep*.[6,35]. The paradigm—to use a word I do not like—of dreaming as half-waking, half-sleeping, persisted.

As I just said, it was by pure chance that in 1958 we stumbled on the problem from a different point of view. We observed that dreaming was neither sleeping nor waking. It was obviously a *third state* of the brain, as different from sleep as sleep is from wakefulness.[76,85,86] *It coincided with paradoxical sleep.*

Much of what we know about this strange state was discovered here in Lyon by students of the Military School of Medicine, the "santards," who were not even paid. Over the years we have been able to analyze paradoxical sleep, and I shall describe those results more fully in later chapters. Suffice it to say now that paradoxical sleep is the periodic appearance during "normal" sleep (so-called *slow wave sleep* because brain electrical activity is relatively slow) of phases of *deep sleep* characterized by brain activity like that of waking, rapid movements of the eyes, and almost complete paralysis of the body's muscles.

A particularly colorful period occurred during the study of *phylogenetic* (the natural history of species in relation to each other) and *ontogenetic* (the natural history of the development of individuals in a given species) aspects of paradoxical sleep. At that time we could buy animals anywhere. If we wished to look at birds we bought a chicken or a goose. We brought in sheep, rabbits, crocodiles, tortoises, a python, iguanas ...

Suddenly, a *unitary* theory of sleep, at least, was overturned. Physiologists had to abandon the very simple "reticular" theory of sleeping and waking and try to reconcile themselves with two new concepts: one was that sleep was an active phenomenon, and the other that there were two states of sleep. This revolution attracted many researchers. Up to about 1985 the field of sleep research was one of the most active in neurophysiology.

So, by 1959, paradoxical sleep had been discovered, and then we showed that an animal could be prevented from sleeping by brain lesions. And in 1969 came the *mono-aminergic* theory of sleep, which lasted for ten years. *Mono-amines* constitute a group of *neurotransmitters* in the brain, the chemical messengers that allow one nerve cell (or *neuron*) to pass information to another. They include some very important substances, which we shall meet later, such as *serotonin* (also called 5-hydroxytryptamine, or 5-HT) and *catecholamines* (including *norepinephrine*).

So began a very fertile period when everything was explained by the neurotransmitters that had just been discovered. The one that interested us at the beginning was acetylcholine. Serotonin came next. Now we know of dozens. But to have dozens is like having none at all. Three or four are enough: one to say "yes," one to say "no," then one for "perhaps yes" and one for "perhaps no." If neuronal systems work in a computer-like way, it is enough. They do not need to be able to say "That is a black chicken" or, "That is a white chicken"! There would never be enough genes for that.

When we realized that neurotransmitters could not explain everything we entered a long period of pessimism. And people who had said, "If you give us money we will explain everything: thought, memory, even mental illness!" saw their grants cut off. In most countries there was a regression of basic physiological research in favor of applied research. In the United States, in Reagan's time, it was no mere coincidence that aging became a principal research topic! Researchers began to record sleep in twenty-year-old cats, which is not a bad age if you consider that you must multiply the age of a cat by six or seven. Because they had to find something, they showed that very old cats had a rather disturbed sleep pattern. There was also much work on *sleep apnea*. People who eat too much, who have short necks, and who snore, stop breathing periodically during sleep, which is bad for the heart if it happens too often.

In France, meanwhile, we must admit that we were accorded great freedom in our research projects. People know very well that sleep is a complicated problem and that dreaming is perhaps the last frontier of neurobiology: we shall certainly understand perception before we understand dreaming. Depending on the amount of money spent, and thus the number of neuroanatomists employed, I think that we could understand just about the whole of the brain's organization within a quarter of a century. But I do not think that we shall have advanced much as far as dreaming is concerned.

When talking about dreams, I like to use the adjective "oneiric" (from the Greek *oneiros*, dream). The problem with oneiric activity is that we are confronted by a phenomenon without function. And that is rare in the annals of physiology. Let me explain. It is very easy to find a small structure in the brain, but more difficult to determine its function. In any case there is no direct relationship between structure and function. We have known that since Claude Bernard. A function implies integrated activity in numerous structures. Take the pineal gland. We took so long to understand its function because we did not integrate it enough. We tried to give it an individual function, whereas it depends on integration with other systems. We now know that it calculates when daytime is lengthening or shortening. If it is shortening, animals should not breed, or they will give birth in winter. It is thus a very important structure in evolution, even if it is less so for us now. It has come back into importance in the last few years, for it secretes a hormone, *melatonin*, which has a profound effect on circadian sleep-wake cycles, and has been promoted in some quarters as a sort of "sleep hormone." We shall come back to melatonin briefly in chapter 8.

But a dream is not the pineal; it is not even a structure! It is something that occupies a fifth of our sleeping time. Dreams are dangerous for an animal because it is paralyzed and its waking threshold is increased. They are *necessary*, for if they are suppressed they tend to return automatically, and the brain tries to make up the lost dream time. Dreams have been conserved throughout evolution, although we still do not know why! I shall try to give a few indicators as to how we may try to understand their function.

We must begin with sleep, which we now know to be related to energy. The human brain spends energy in thinking, in a similar way to a working muscle. It is rather like an experimental proof of the subconscious adage that "thinking is tiring!" Between phases of rest and phases of intense brain activity the consumption of energy-giving sugar (*glucose*) in the cerebral cortex (the thin outer layer of the brain that deals with "higher" nervous activity) doubles without change in oxygen uptake. This means that our brain can work against an oxygen "debt". When it does, it produces *lactate*, a chemical characteristic of such *anaerobic* metabolism: it "tires" like working muscles, which also produce lactate.[49] The neurotransmitters that keep us awake break down molecules of *glycogen*, the form in which glucose is commonly stored in the body as an energy reserve. Sleep must intervene to allow the brain to replenish its stocks of energy, mainly in the *glial cells*, the non-nervous "support" cells of the brain responsible for its protection and nourishment.[89] Its temperature also falls.[57] In man a fall in temperature of 1 °C takes about ninety minutes. Then, and only then, strange systems—perhaps thermoreceptors sensitive to a hundredth of a degree—alert the brain that energy reserves have been replenished (see below). Another detection system is based on the so-called *redox potential*, a physiological signal that is related to the aspects of energy metabolism that rely on the use of oxygen. It indicates to the part of the brain that controls dreams that enough energy, in the form of the common energy storage molecule adenosine triphosphate (*ATP*), has been accumulated. Then a dream comes on, spending a large amount of energy, before another long period of energy accumulation starts. We are beginning to understand how all this works. It still remains for us to discover the system that enables the brain to sense its energy levels, which will certainly be more sophisticated than the systems we are studying at present.

The regulation of paradoxical sleep by temperature is very surprising because it does not respect certain well-established biological rules, such as the laws of van't Hoff and Arrhenius according to which the speed of a chemical reaction decreases when the temperature falls. A relationship called $Q_{10}$ (the temperature coefficient) exists between the activity of a system (respiration, heart rate, oxygen consumption, and many others) at 37 °C (the normal body temperature for many animals) and 10 °C lower (at 27 °C). This relationship is always between 2 and 3. This means that a decrease in temperature of 10 °C causes an approximate halving in the activity of biological systems. However, regulation of paradoxical sleep seems doubly paradoxical: on the one hand the amount of paradoxical sleep *increases* tenfold when body temperature decreases by 10 °C, such that the $Q_{10}$ is 0.1, and on the other hand paradoxical sleep itself triggers a cooling system. An open loop with no feedback thus exists: the more body temperature falls, the more paradoxical sleep increases and the more the temperature falls. It looks as if the "aim" of this system is to obtain permanent paradoxical sleep at about 20 °C.

Obviously there are several possible models that could explain these phenomena. The simplest model depends on thermoreceptors in the brain. Some of them are stimulated by heat—and they could be the arousal systems (blockers of paradoxical sleep). Others are stimulated by cold, and we could assume that they trigger paradoxical sleep. Nevertheless this hypothesis is not very robust, for we must assume that we warm-blooded animals (whose temperature is always above about 35 °C) have nerve cells that work best between 25° and 20 °C (the temperature of our cold-blooded predecessors a few million years ago). This would mean that dinosaur thermoreceptors still exist in our brain. But why not?

The idea of *thermoreceptors* is now being elaborated into one of *thermostats*, capable of maintaining a constant body temperature. But, by definition, a thermostat has a negative feedback loop, which is not the case with our dream system, which is an open loop with no feedback. So a third model is possible. It depends on cerebral energy levels, which implies knowing the consumption of both glucose and oxygen when the temperature falls from 37° to 27 °C.

So, we really must tackle the problem of cerebral energy. For years this proved an obstacle that was impenetrable for technical reasons. New techniques are often needed in order to advance in physiology, and they are beginning to appear. We now have the *positron emission tomography* camera (or *PET scanner*). This device allows us to visualize the consumption of glucose and oxygen in the living human brain, enabling "maps" of cortical activity to be constructed on the basis of local changes in energy and blood flow, something that we never succeeded in doing before. In experimental animals, spectroscopic magnetic resonance imaging (rather like the revolutionary MRI scanner used in human medical imaging) gives us the possibility of seeing energy sources, such as peaks of ATP, without touching the brain—a marvelous achievement. We can also use the so-called *deoxyglucose* method. This is rather similar to PET scanning, except that it involves injection of a special form of radioactive glucose and the study of slices of the brain after death. This means, again, that it is an experimental technique, rather than a clinical one. So in the next few years we are going to be able to take positive steps in directions in which no progress has been made for a good twenty years or more. This in turn may enable us to decide whether transmitters or energy is all-important.

So energy holds a secret somewhere. In order to make progress we need physiologists capable of a synthetic view of the various highly complex mechanisms involved in energy transformation and in communication between neurons and, undoubtedly, between neurons and glia. This is why I plead for the sort of physiology that we are slowly allowing to disappear. We must realize that, throughout the world, the proportion of basic physiological research involved in international study of sleep and dreaming dropped from 60% in 1960 to 10% in 1996! Things are similar in all countries. We shall soon find ourselves with large numbers of molecular biologists who have absolutely no idea of how the organism functions! I like to imagine not the twilight of molecular biology—because it has contributed so much and provided an extraordinarily rich harvest—but rather its relative deemphasis, at least in relation to the central nervous system, so that it may give way to other approaches, particularly energy studies. But I do not believe this will happen on its own. At the moment molecular biologists are particularly vigilant in maintaining their position at all costs. We have already seen an explosion of brain models based on the molecular biology of *receptors*, the protein molecules located in membranes of cells that enable specific chemicals, including neurotransmitters, to act on those cells.

Another tendency, based on computer studies, will also probably turn into a flood: this concerns models of machines with *artificial intelligence*, and perhaps even thought! In my opinion, comparing the brain to a computer is a deceptive metaphor that disregards brain development during ontogeny and cerebral *plasticity* (the capacity of the brain to change its fine structure to improve its efficiency, especially by adapting to environmental pressures). Above all it neglects the fact that a computer runs on electricity, and therefore has no energy problems, whereas the brain must control its own energy requirements, as well as those of the organism. Once again, I would be really interested in knowing how these models take account of sleeping and dreaming.

However, I too, like many others, have contributed to slowing down progress. For instance, for many years I believed that serotonin was responsible for sleep. At the time, my students put up a photograph of Mao waving his *Little Red Book* as a joke. Now I know that the problem is much more complex and I have abandoned the idea that a single factor is adequate to trigger a dream. The cause of sleep or dreams is really an ensemble of conditions, but one is tempted to think that the last condition is the cause. That is why this type of research is so slow. Various obstacles to progress must be eliminated, obstacles that are often created by powerful groups that publish a lot. For example, in the mid-1960s the dogma persisted that oxygen consumption by the brain did not vary between sleeping and waking. We now know that there was a statistical error in those results, but it still led to most researchers avoiding the energy theme.

Thus one of the probable keys to the mechanism of dreaming is that it needs a lot of energy. Another key is provided by phylogenesis. Why is there such a difference between *cold-blooded* animals—lower vertebrates, which do not regulate their temperature—and *warm-blooded* animals, which maintain a constant temperature independent of outside conditions? No one has yet recorded with certainty a state similar to paradoxical sleep in fish, amphibians, and reptiles, except perhaps in the crocodile. Why, then, have fish not needed to invent paradoxical sleep? How do we explain this enigma? I think one answer lies in *neurogenesis*, the "birth" of neurons by cell division. In cold-blooded animals, neurons divide throughout their whole life. Some brain cells of a sixty-year-old carp are still dividing! In contrast, after about 21 days in rats and cats, and from midgestation in man, neurons stop dividing and only have one fate: death. We shall come back to this in chapter 7.

A third key is provided by ontogenesis, which brings us two concepts. The more immature a mammal or bird just before or just after birth, the more it has something like paradoxical sleep (which we call *active* sleep, as opposed to *quiet* sleep, the equivalent in the immature brain to slow wave sleep). It ends with the end of the genetic programming of the brain, at the end of neurogenesis. It is not really paradoxical sleep because it

cannot be suppressed by drugs or lesions that suppress paradoxical sleep in the adult. As soon as neurogenesis stops,
true paradoxical sleep appears, accompanied by a range of
apparently aimless facial expressions and real smiles in human
babies, and the idea of a program emerges.

What is the use of such a program? I think the case of twins
may help to explain. If we consider twins raised completely
apart since birth, of course, no one will be surprised that they
look alike. But Tom Bouchard at the University of Minnesota
found much stranger things by studying dozens of pairs of
identical twins brought up since birth in different families. How
can we explain the extraordinarily similar events that occurred
during their lives? (see chapter 7). How can we explain their
psychological heredity, responsible for their identical idiosyncratic reactions even when they had been subjected to different
experiences and environments during their whole life?

If nerve cell division continued throughout life (*continuous
neurogenesis*) we could imagine that the genetic program in
their DNA might preserve an identical psychological patrimony
in each twin. But this cannot happen, for the central nervous
system is unique in the body in that its principal cells, the
neurons, cannot divide in adult life. So do we have to accept
that the genetic program active during prenatal and immediate
postnatal development is responsible once and for all for the
myriad subtle interneuronal connections that cause our various
character traits throughout life? That is simply impossible.
First, genetic programming of the thousands of billions of
*synapses* (the connections between one neuron and the next)
would need a far greater number of genes than contained in the
whole genome. Second, the influence of the environment would
ultimately change these connections through the process of
neuronal plasticity, mentioned above.

So can we conceive of genetic programs being periodically reinforced in order to maintain the functional synaptic circuits responsible for psychological heredity? The advantage of such a system would obviously be that it could permit the reestablishment of any circuits that had been altered by events not under direct genetic control (*epigenetic* events). My hypothesis is that this genetic reprogramming occurs during paradoxical sleep, that is, during dreaming.

But why? Well, simply to restore individuality. For diversity is extremely important. And above all it is very important that, in a conditioning environment such as ours, we have access to a system that preserves individuality.

We are at this very moment living out the historic failure of attempts to change man by changing the environment. Heaven knows how much propaganda has been poured out and people shot to convince others to think properly! So why has it failed? Perhaps because people have continued to dream. What did the KGB do with dissenters? They put them in psychiatric hospitals. Why? Among other things, they gave them drugs that suppressed dreams, such as those called phenothiazine derivatives or monoamine oxidase inhibitors. They presumably knew that people on these drugs, who therefore dreamed less or not at all, became more easily conditioned to accept the ideological environment.

This hypothesis of the repeated reprogramming of individuality during dreaming (see chapter 7) is not very well appreciated by the scientific intelligentsia. Psychological inheritance is seen as dubious since Théodule-Armand Ribot's exaggerated claims relating memory and evolution. Current dogma is that our psychological profile depends on cultural environment and changing it can "improve" an individual. As soon as one speaks of psychological inheritance or individuality people think of the old debate on intelligence, IQ, and social class. This has nothing to do with my hypothesis.

I encountered resistance on two occasions when I wanted to try to tackle the problem in man. We had discovered that different strains of mice (the only animal that dreams in which we can easily study genetic aspects of paradoxical sleep by breeding specific strains) present characteristic REM patterns during paradoxical sleep[21]: some strains show much movement, others very little. Furthermore, the strains with little movement proved more "intelligent" in maze tests than those with much movement .

This observation led us to explore possible difference between patterns of eye movements during dreaming in human groups differing genetically in that they were what are termed *genetic isolates*. In 1972, thanks to the courtesy and generosity of Professor Robert Gessain and his wife from the Musée de l'Homme in Paris, we went to record sleep of the Bassaris—a people already well studied genetically—who live in the bush between Senegal and Guinea. This little expedition made a change from our laboratory routine: we had to transport an EEG machine, a small computer to record eye movements, and batteries, and we had to make our recordings in the Bassaris' huts after long palavers to obtain the permission of the women. I have happy memories of the nights, fortunately quite cool, spent recording four adult male Bassaris surrounded by the sounds of the bush. In spite of many difficulties we managed to record about twenty periods of sleep and we were immediately struck by the rarity of eye movements during these periods. I shall not go into details about our daytime activities when we became doctors treating dozens of Bassaris or Fulani suffering from conditions that you only find in old medical dictionaries, while a dentist took out the few filed-off teeth of the old folk. I shall also spare you the dances, the buffalo sacrifice, collecting honey from trees, tracking lions, and much more.

Thanks to the great experience of the ethnologists and their knowledge of the Bassaris, we were able to bring two of our subjects to Lyon. After they had been in France for a few months we again recorded them in our laboratory and still found a significant difference in the frequency and pattern of their eye movements compared with a control population. So we submitted a short note to an international scientific journal. Our very prudent conclusion was that there could be significant, perhaps genetic, differences between different human groups. Our note was rejected both because the number of subjects was too small (I agree) and because the demonstration of fewer eye movements in Bassaris was interpreted in an unfavorable, or even racist, light!

In spite of this first experience, and thanks to a friend who was a connoisseur of the Far North, I tried to study another much less isolated and colorful population: the Laplanders. So, letters to embassies, to the scientific attaché in Norway to explain the aims of our visit, and so on. Finally the Laplanders learned of our project. One day I received a letter with a magnificent heading proclaiming the decolonization of arctic nations, including the Laplanders, the Eskimos, and the Nenets, or Samoyeds. The letter was insulting: we would be "collecting data from foreign cultures," indulging in "physical anthropology ... a thing of the past," risking "frightening consequences (racially conditioned determinism)." There was no question of Laplanders serving as subjects for experiments. I replied that, on the contrary, if we managed to show that their eye movement patterns during dreaming were different from those of Norwegians it could provide them with an additional argument for claiming independence. For once oneirological research might make a positive contribution! The reply was unequivocal: if we came we would be met with guns. There was no way that I was going to die for ethno-oneirology! We therefore used the modest (private) funding for our mission to do some cod fishing off the Lofoten Islands. This too left happy memories of late winter, fog, gray seas, and grilled cod tongues with brandy ...

I regret that I was not able to pursue this work. Human groups disappear every day without our being able to record the pattern of their eye movements during dreaming. Even if we do not *yet* know how to decipher their dream code (can we call them *oneiremes?*), it may be possible one day, and this treasure will be lost forever. Who knows what fundamental facts about man's origins they might have revealed? I spoke about the urgency of such ethno-oneirological studies at a conference in Kyoto, but I do not think they understood what I meant.

Finally, because I am stubborn, as a solid Franche-Comté man tends to be, we undertook a third attempt in Lyon on ten pairs of identical and nonidentical twins. We recorded on tape tens of thousands of eye movements during dreaming. At the time, in 1976, we had no personal computers, so one of my students, Guy Chouvet—experienced in information technology and mathematics—spent thousands of hours analyzing the results. He spent four years using some of the biggest computers of that time. His superb thesis showed the similarity of patterns in identical twins, whereas there is none in nonidentical twins.[24,25] Since then, this excellent researcher has avoided twins and moved into cutting-edge electrophysiology.

To finish the subject of genetics and dreams, I should like to tell you the following story, which is quite genuine. At a reception I had the occasion to speak about memories of dreams to a colleague, a member of the Academy. "When I was a child," he told me, "I often had the same dream: I was passing in front of a big house and I saw a lady dressed in black opening the door of a long corridor." Just at that moment, his twin brother, his spitting image, came up to us and heard the last few words of the story, which he went on to complete spontaneously: "The lady opened the door of the corridor and hundreds of cats ran out." His brother, the academician, looked at him in great surprise. "How could you have finished my dream? I never told you about it."

These twins had had the same dream. It is perhaps a unique case but, nonetheless, exploration of memories of dreams of identical and nonidentical twins could become a very interesting research field, but certainly difficult and very long.

The complexity of the brain and the mechanisms of paradoxical sleep are such that I do not think it will be possible to verify the hypothesis of repeated genetic reprogramming for a long time. Fortunately there are other hypotheses and thus bases for discussion. For instance, a few years ago, I was invited to spend a month at the Salk Institute in California by Francis Crick (codiscoverer of the double helix of DNA). Crick is a very polite man, sometimes charming, sometimes extravagant, and, although now a molecular biologist, has never forgotten his training as a physicist. With an information technologist friend, Crick had elaborated a hypothesis of the function of dreams, for no unknown frontiers can resist either molecular biological or British imperialism! According to his hypothesis, the efficiency of a supercomputer, and therefore a brain, necessitates the periodic appearance of random signals in order to delete memories saturated with insignificant events. This metaphor seems pertinent because in a dream the brain is invaded by random activity. What is more, such programming or deleting operations imply "disconnection" of the "inputs" and "outputs" of the computer. This could be the case during dreaming, because a system of inhibition blocks the entry of signals from the environment and inhibits movements at the level of the motor neurons, except for eye movements and respiration. Crick's hypothesis was, then, that dreams delete unimportant memories. This is the "excretion" hypothesis already proposed in 1886 by Robert,[133] cited by Freud in *The Interpretation of Dreams*.[52] Francis Crick did not know this reference of which I politely reminded him. But we could not find Robert's book in San Diego.

We therefore had long, very lively discussions, both feeling that our theories were contradictory, or at least in part, as my hypothesis could very easily imply the wiping out of certain circuits. We tried to find a way to test Crick's hypothesis. According to him, there should be a correlation between the volume of the cerebral cortex—the memory to delete—and the amount of paradoxical sleep. But I pointed out an exception: the dolphin's cortex is almost as developed as man's but has no paradoxical sleep, as Lev Mukhametov[113,114] had more or less convinced me when I met him in Moscow. This was an enigma, but a Soviet enigma ... As we were near San Diego, where there is an important naval base at which work is carried out on dolphins, we thought they might have studied their sleep. We therefore contacted their research director, a U.S. Navy admiral. Neither Crick's British passport nor my French one was good enough: top secret research, no visiting!

Absence of proof is not proof of absence, concluded Crick, who wrote an article in *Nature*[27] on his theory of *reverse learning*. There are a number of objections to it, even if one forgets the case of the dolphin and even admits that the cat, which dreams twice as much as man, is a special case. The most important objection is that hundreds of depressed patients have been treated with monoamine oxidase inhibitors or tricyclic antidepressants. These drugs suppress paradoxical sleep and dreaming completely, or almost completely, as proved in recordings of their sleep using a *polygraph*. This machine records several physical variables at the same time, such as electrical activity in muscle (the *electromyogram*, or EMG) and brain (the EEG), and has become an essential part of any laboratory devoted to sleep research. But suppression of dreaming for weeks or months has never led to memory loss. This observation is enough to negate the hypothesis of reverse learning. The absence of disturbance of memory or thought processes by these pharmacological means, however, does not negate *my* hypothesis. Frank or subtle changes of personality in someone treated with dream-suppressing antidepressants could certainly be attributed to the disappearance of repetitive genetic reprogramming. But, of course, one can object that the appearance or disappearance of subtle idiosyncratic psychological traits could well be due either to the drugs themselves or to curing the depression. Nevertheless, I do not believe it right to give drugs that suppress dreaming to normal subjects, as was done formerly in the USSR.

I shall now return to the subject of the lack of paradoxical sleep in the dolphin. I respect and admire the work of my friend Lev Mukhametov and his pupils.[113,114] It is not easy to record from dolphins, and the Russians have perfected systems for signal transmission through seawater that work remarkably well. I have seen excellent polygraph traces in Moscow. Whatever the explanation of this mystery, the possible absence of dreaming in dolphins led me to make an unforgettable journey.

In the early 1980s the results of some experiments indicated to us that chemicals called *peptides*, small molecules composed of amino acids and secreted from the pituitary gland (see figure

1), could considerably increase paradoxical sleep in the cat. For a number of years I even supposed, wrongly, that these substances were both *necessary* and *adequate* to cause paradoxical sleep. We managed to show that peptides could act either directly via a nerve pathway between the hypothalamus (the part of the brain that controls pituitary function) and the brainstem—where the "machinery" of paradoxical sleep lies— or via the bloodstream after liberation from the pituitary. Lev Mukhametov had sent us two dolphin brains. Thanks to our excellent team of immunohistochemists, mainly Japanese, we were able to demonstrate that the organization of certain peptide systems in the dolphin was different from that in the cat. We wondered if an "oneirogenic" peptide or peptides were present in the pituitary of the dolphin. To test this, we had to get some, which is easier said than done! There are only two places in the world where fishermen still deliberately kill dolphins, in Turkey and in Japan, where they cause considerable damage by destroying fishing nets along the coast. So I set off, for the tenth time, to Japan, and on to Okinawa. Thanks to the extraordinary efficiency of the Japanese we were soon in possession of a dozen or so pituitaries, stored in large thermos flasks filled with dry ice.

It was then that we learned that a new strain of cat had been discovered at Iriomote, the southernmost island of the Ryukyu archipelago, 80 miles east of Taiwan. It is a small island, so covered with mangroves that it was spared by the war. The sand is composed of tiny starlike fragments of coral, and the flora and fauna are unique. There was a population of fifty or so cats with six toes, which did not purr, and spent their time in the water eating fish. These cats were studied and protected by the same number of Japanese researchers and were so precious that we soon gave up the idea of asking to record their sleep and dreams. In fact we never saw the cats of Iriomote, but we spent some unforgettable days on this sun-drenched island, which was still utterly devoid of tourists.

We returned to Lyon with our dolphin pituitaries. But our original hypothesis was flawed. We now know, thanks to a group in another laboratory, that the increase in sleep provoked by hypothalamic peptides is a response to stress due to deprivation of paradoxical sleep (see chapter 7), thus demonstrating that these peptides are *neither* necessary *nor* adequate to trigger dreams, but can be responsible for pathological oversleeping (hypersomnia).

This story of the dolphins gives an idea of how "cutting-edge" this research on the neurobiological mechanisms of dreams was. Dreaming, as I have said, is one of the last frontiers of neuroscience. We still, I am happy to say, have one foot in the eighteenth century with our continued effort to study the natural history of dreaming throughout evolution. However, for reasons of scientific credibility we must have the other foot in biochemistry, looking for *the* oneiric molecule, although I no longer believe there is one since I abandoned the idea of necessary and adequate causality. Indeed, some current concepts based on molecular biology or genetics make me think of the Lego that my children played with. In spite of its complexity, the extraordinary fascination of an energy-based approach to the alternation of waking-sleeping-dreaming stems from the possibility that it might resolve the problem of mechanism as well as of function. This approach is unfortunately absent from molecular biological and neural network models.

I believe that we shall need much time, and generations of researchers, to understand how the brain regulates its energy and that of the whole organism. This is why it is difficult for me to write a book on the physiology of waking, sleeping, and dreaming. Furthermore, I think that my generation of sleep researchers have spent our allotted time rather blindly. We rather unwisely stayed awake day and night for years in a frantic and exhausting race to try to understand a phenomenon that had suddenly become finite, quantifiable, and of which we believed we could probe the function.

Of course I do not regret the years between 1960 and 1980, the sleepless nights at the hospital, in the laboratory, or in airplanes. But I believe that our mistake was to believe that research into mechanisms, structures, and neurotransmitters would lead us to function or functions. The problem is that we progressed from one neurotransmitter, acetylcholine, to serotonin, and now know of dozens! We seem to add some more every week. Was our strategy wrong? Probably. But definitely wrong in time management, because time has become too short now to integrate the immense capital of experimental data amassed in "old" laboratories like those of William Dement in Stanford, Allen Rechtschaffen in Chicago, Howard Roffwarg in Dallas, and in others, some of which have already disappeared. Most of this data were acquired before the advent of microcomputers. The "memories" of many experiments—unique, unreproducible, and therefore unpublishable—are stored in, and are slowly being deleted from, our sexagenarian brains. They sometimes come back to us during the evening at conferences, in an American or Japanese bar, but these memories are difficult to transfer to the younger generation.

It was presumptuous to believe it was possible to resolve the mystery of the mechanisms and functions of dreams in the forty years that we have had access to objective criteria. To understand dream consciousness is indeed the last frontier of neurobiology—beyond even our understanding of waking consciousness. Can we even tell if the conscious brain will one day be able to explain why it is conscious of being conscious?

Searching for curiosity's sake, looking for what is behind an obstacle, is genetically programmed behavior, as we can see by studying strains of mice. So, maybe one of the functions of dreams in some people is to program the idea that there might exist an answer to an insoluble problem—that of the function of dreams ...

# 2

## The Natural History of Dreaming

Dreams are subjective phenomena that only become realities if we can remember their contents after waking.

How many of you remember your dreams? About 80% according to the statistics. But the 20% who think they do not dream can be reassured, for they do in fact dream every night, but the moment they wake they wipe out the memory of their oneiric activity. This is perhaps because their waking brain has forgotten the scenario of their dream, or its action, or cannot accept it. I hope the story of dreaming that I am now going to recount briefly will convince you that the machinery of dreaming always functions periodically in our brains while we sleep.

### The Metaphysical Theory of Dreaming

Dreams were once attributed to messages from gods or demons. Now we try to explain their contents in psychological terms. Some forty years ago they became part of the neurobiology of warm-blooded vertebrates.

This long history stretches back to the origins of man. I wonder how long it was before this nightly repetition of

Originally published in 1981 in the series *Dialogues—Le Cerveau en Images*, INSERM *and Palais de la Découverte.*

fantastic imagery led him to the essential conclusion that marked the dawn of humanity? That some immaterial element, some "spirit" or "soul" must exist, fundamentally different from the material body, an untiring and invisible spirit *that stays awake during sleep*. It wanders freely though space and time and delivers oneiric images of its voyage to the brain while the tired body is deep in sleep. *Soul* implies immortality, which requires burial of the body. So, according to James Lovelock, to Herbert Spencer, and to Bronislaw Malinowski, the fantastic nature of dreams was at the origin of belief in the spirit and the soul that we find in various forms at the dawn of all civilizations and in all religions.

The metaphysical side of dreams still persists today. The fellahs of the Nile delta envelop their head with a turban to prevent their soul escaping from their skull during sleep, and the Masai of Kenya do not wake a sleeper suddenly for fear that his wandering spirit may not be able to reenter his body.

The dreams of prophets can be related to this metaphysical trend: the dreams of Jacob, or the Pharaoh, and of Nebuchadnezzar in the Old Testament; the dreams of Joseph, the magi, and during the flight into Egypt in the New Testament. Of course, the founders of religious orders must have had a privileged relationship with God through dreams. So it was with Macaire of Egypt, St. Francis of Assisi, Don Bosco, St. Bruno. Equally, warriors could only vanquish through the oracle of dreams: witness Xerxes in his campaign in Greece and many others!

Looking into the future is a basic process of the human mind. That is why we note the success of dreambooks and interpreters of dreams since the time of Artemidore of Ephesus and the cabalistic tradition.

## Psychological Theories of Dreaming

Just as the metaphysical trend was losing its inertia, another trend, this time psychological, was growing. It became interested in the relationship of dreams, still considered as a timeless phenomenon during sleep, with memory and consciousness, and with stimuli outside sleep.

This psychological trend was initiated by Aristotle, who considered sleep as simply activity of the mind during sleep (with no question of communication with God), and grew at the end of the eighteenth century and during the nineteenth. It is impossible to cite here all the different theories of sleep that saw the light of day. For some, sensations from our limbs and other external or internal stimuli were the sources of the hallucinations of the sleeper. Henri Bergson believed that dream images were due to intrinsic retinal images.

Gradually the fashion of studying one's own dreams grew in the scientific community. Competitions took place in different learned academies. Yves Delage, already well known for his controversies with Darwin on heredity, wrote daily accounts of his dreams in his laboratory in Roscoff in Brittany.[31] He noted that he had no dream recollection of the declaration of war in 1914, nor of the death of certain persons close to him. Analyzing his memories in detail, he formulated the hypothesis that the repressed "psyche" of the waking state appeared in dreams. This idea of *repression* had already been formulated 25 years earlier by Robert[133] for whom dreams were the manifestations of thoughts "stifled at birth."

So many names cropped up during this period that it would take hours to draw up the list. Some of the personalities who have studied dreaming are quite strange themselves. For instance, Hervey de Saint-Denis, professor of Chinese at the Collège de France, claimed to be able to direct his dreams, which I think is quite exceptional. On the other hand, *lucid* dreams are now in fashion and the center of media attention. They are dreams in which we are aware of our presence in a dream, and have a limited influence on their enactment. Hervey de Saint-Denis' book contains a masterful history of psychological theories of dreaming: *Nihil est in visionibus somniorum quod not prius fuerit in visu,* he wrote, insisting on the importance of childhood memories and of their repression.

It is odd that Freud did not read Hervey de Saint-Denis' book and never evoked the problems of the time course of dreams within sleep. Freud, inventor of metapsychology, rejects everything to do with sleep because it is physiology. Freud considered dreaming as the expression of repressed wishes and the *guardian of sleep.* He imagined a veritable psychic apparatus *outside* the brain. This topic brings us to consider the space corresponding to the *id,* the *ego,* and the *superego,* concepts that made their mark and still await their impossible experimental refuting.

We shall end this review of the psychological trend with Jung. His unconscious differs from Freud's in that it is supposedly the seat of universal primordial images common to all civilizations. For instance the dream of a phallic sun goes back to the cult of Mithras.

## The Temporal Structure of Dreams

Since the end of the nineteenth century, dreams have acquired a temporal structure. This second direction for exploration was of utmost importance, for it predicted modern neurobiology.

Alfred Maury woke sleeping subjects at regular intervals and noted that they only rarely recalled dreams. This refuted the concept of dreaming occurring permanently during sleep. For Maury, dreaming was an episodic or random phenomenon appearing when sleep was lightest, either during the process of falling asleep (*hypnagogic* images), or under the influence of stimuli outside the body (such as noise), or inside it (such as pain), or just before waking (*hypnopompic* images). The phenomenon of dreaming thus became related to the *type* of sleep and its interaction with waking. It lost its timeless character and began to become physiological. Alfred Maury is equally famous for his dream of the guillotine, which is often cited, but this is apocryphal for it was written more than fifty years later.

The work of Henri Piéron is of great historical importance even if it does not concern dreaming directly. In 1913 Piéron managed to transfer "hypnotoxins" from the blood or ventricles of a dog that was deprived of sleep to a recipient and to induce a state of deep sleep in it. Piéron's work has been much criticized, especially by Raphaël Dubois of Lyon, the man who described carbon dioxide narcosis and luciferine, and Edouard Claparède of Geneva for whom sleep was an instinct, and it fell into oblivion. It has reemerged since the discovery of certain chemicals that "facilitate" sleep. The hypothesis of a factor or factors being responsible for sleeping and dreaming is now the subject of numerous projects.

## The Neurobiological Basis of Dreaming

Since 1880 a neurobiological basis for dreaming has slowly taken shape, like the pieces of a puzzle. In 1880 Jean-Baptiste

Gélineau, a former naval physician, described *narcolepsy* (Gélineau's syndrome).[55] Without realizing it he described one of the fundamental characteristics of dreaming, the almost total absence of muscular tone. Narcolepsy, which can also affect dogs and ponies, is relatively common in man. It presents as the sudden and irremediable onset of sleep, or as a loss of muscle tone following some emotion such as hearty laughter, leading to a fall. These *cataplectic attacks* are often accompanied by dreams and the subject loses touch with the reality of the outside world. In rare cases the subject remains conscious because only the system for postural atonia, the loss of tone in the body's main muscles, is triggered.

It can readily be understood that drugs aimed at controlling narcolepsy might prevent paradoxical sleep. This is the case of some antidepressants, like monoamine oxidase inhibitors and tricyclics, which, by raising the concentration of serotonin or catecholamines (such as norepinephrine), block the appearance of paradoxical sleep.

Little by little in the course of the first half of the twentieth century the pieces of the puzzle of dreaming were gathered. In 1937 Klaue described periods of deep sleep in the cat accompanied by fast electrical activity in the cerebral cortex very different from the normal slow cortical activity of sleep. His work was forgotten. In 1944 another German, Ohlmeyer,[117] described a periodic cycle of penile erections in men during sleep. The cycle started 90 minutes after falling asleep, and the phases of erection were twenty-five minutes long on average, with an average periodicity of eighty-five minutes. These times correspond to the periodicity of dreaming, but erection was not seen as related to dreams at the time (figure 2).

Loss of muscle function during narcolepsy, periodic erection, and fast cortical activity—these pathognomonic signs of

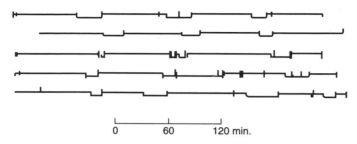

**Figure 2**
Tracing of the cycle of penile erection during five different nights. There are three to four periods of erection each night (downward trace). Each erection starts about sixty to ninety minutes after falling asleep and their distribution during the night is similar to that of dreams. (From Ohlmeyer et al.[117])

dreaming were thus almost all available in 1944, but were not integrated. It had taken almost seventy years, since 1880, to assemble them. The history of science teaches us that, for a discipline to be productive, it must interact with others at both the conceptual and technical levels. Science cannot be reduced to a single statement: it must be interdisciplinary. How then can we hope to understand a highly integrated phenomenon like dreaming from molecular biology alone?

We saw in chapter 1 that in 1953 Eugene Aserinsky delivered the last piece of the puzzle by discovering rapid eye movement (REM) sleep. His hypothesis was that this might correspond to periods of dreaming. Then, between 1953 and 1957, William Dement and Nathaniel Kleitman put the puzzle together, but backward.[34] They woke subjects during REM sleep on 191 occasions. In 152, or 80%, they recalled dreams very clearly. In contrast, they woke subjects during slow wave sleep 160 times and only got 11 reports of dreams (7%). Dreams occurred for periods of twenty to twenty-five minutes separated by intervals of ninety minutes. For the Chicago

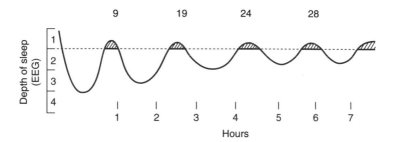

**Figure 3**
The concept of the Chicago school. The depth of sleep is represented on the abscissa. The periods of dreaming (with their duration indicated in minutes) represent a stage of light sleep (emergent stage 1) similar to falling asleep (descending stage 1).

school, then, dreaming was considered as a periodic phase of light sleep (*emergent stage 1*), analogous to falling asleep (*descending stage 1*) (figures 3 and 4).

As we have already seen, the puzzle was finally put together the right way in 1959 thanks to animal neurophysiology which put dreaming in its proper place in the cycle of waking and sleeping.[75,76,77] Throughout the ages, since Aristotle, hunters have noticed that their dogs sometimes move while they are asleep. But it was thanks to the cat that dreams entered the neurophysiological arena. Polygraphic study of sleep-wake cycles by electrodes implanted chronically in various major brain structures and in different muscle groups enabled us to explore the two quite different components of sleep, as I already mentioned briefly in chapter 1. One was *slow wave sleep*, accompanied by slow, high-amplitude cortical electrical waves, and normal muscle tone. The other was a deep sleep, characterized paradoxically by brain activity similar to that of waking, by rapid eye movements, and by almost total loss of muscle tone (figure 5). This is the sleep state that I named *par-*

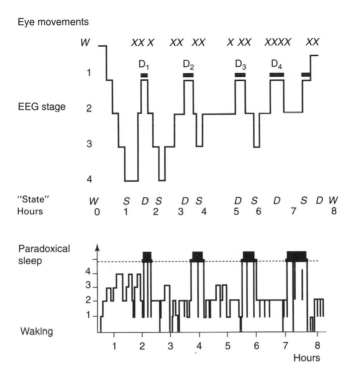

**Figure 4**
Schematic diagram of a normal night's sleep (hypnogram) to illustrate different theories of sleep. Top: For some, dreams ($D_1$–$D_4$) are included in stage 1 (light sleep). W, waking; S, sleep. Middle: Paradoxical sleep is represented, in heavy black, as deeper than the deepest sleep (stage 4). This is my concept.

*adoxical sleep* (see chapter 1). It lasts for about five minutes and happens every twenty-five minutes during sleep in the cat (figure 6).

Very soon we noticed that loss of muscle tone also occurred in man and that human dreaming and paradoxical sleep in the cat had the same neurobiological basis, at least in physiological terms. There was no way that dreaming could be considered

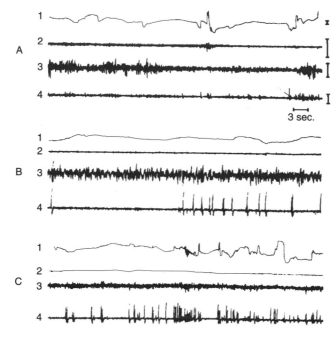

**Figure 5**
Polygraph recordings of the three stages of vigilance in the cat:
A, waking; B, normal sleep; C, paradoxical sleep. Record 1 shows
rapid eye movements. Record 2: electromyogram of the neck muscles.
Record 3: cortical activity. Record 4: activity in the lateral geniculate
nucleus, where PGO activity appears during paradoxical sleep. The
cortical recordings during waking and paradoxical sleep are identical.
This is why muscle activity must be recorded to detect paradoxical
sleep.

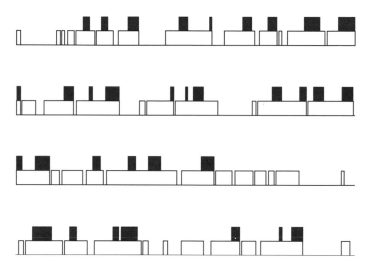

**Figure 6**
Paradoxical sleep is a periodic phenomenon. In the cat it occurs every
25 minutes during sleep. Each line covers four hours of recording. The
black blocks represent paradoxical sleep, the white blocks are slow
wave sleep, and the intervening periods are waking. The periodicity of
paradoxical sleep seems proportional to the logarithm of the weight of
an animal (7 minutes in the mouse, 90 minutes in the human, 180
minutes in the elephant). The precise nature of the ultradian pacemaker responsible for this periodicity is unknown.

any longer as light sleep. *Dreaming became the third state of
the brain, as different from sleep as sleep was from waking.*

The idea of dreaming as a third state of the brain is merely
a new form of an age-old concept—that of the Upanishads
of Hindu mythology—according to which the human brain
alternates between waking, sleeping without dreams, and sleeping with dreams.

Neurobiologists certainly did not *need* a third state of cerebral function. Indeed, an alternation of waking and sleeping is

a priori enough to explain the alternation of "activity" and "rest" in our brain cells, at least in those responsible for higher nervous activity.

Faced with the discovery of these new horizons in the brain, neurophysiology adopted two attitudes to try to find an explanation of dreaming. One was global, looking for the natural history of the phenomenon: when did it begin in phylogenetic or ontogenetic evolution? The other was reductionist: what do we know of the neurobiological mechanisms of paradoxical sleep? In other words, can we deduce the function of dreaming from its structures and its mechanisms?

In man, a night's sleep consists of a succession of different stages, usually numbered from 1 to 4, corresponding to increasingly slow electrical activity in the cerebral cortex (hence the name slow wave sleep, as I explained earlier). The different stages of slow wave sleep are not accompanied by eye movements, but some of the muscle tone found in waking remains. If you wake a sleeper during slow wave sleep he rarely remembers dreaming (see figure 4 and chapter 3).

We have already seen how the phases of slow wave sleep are interrupted by the appearance of another phase characterized by fast cortical activity, rapid eye movements, and an almost total loss of muscle tone (*postural atonia*). A few discrete movements of the face, like traces of a smile or a grimace, or of the fingers, can sometimes persist, but organized limb movements are very rare. The Chicago school of Nathaniel Kleitman, Eugene Aserinsky, and William Dement proved that subjects woken at this stage could relate their dreams in great detail. It was possible in some cases to correlate the direction of eye movements with scenes encountered in dreams, and this gave rise to the hypothesis that the eye movements could be a reflection of visual exploration of the dream world, scanning the scene or looking at it attentively. We shall come back to this later. This state has been given various names by different schools, not only REM sleep or paradoxical sleep but also desynchronized sleep, dreaming state, D state, and others (see the Lexicon). I must again emphasize that dreaming is accompanied by total postural atonia, so sleepwalking, for example, does not belong to dream activity, but represents an incomplete awakening during stages 3 or 4 of slow wave sleep.

The study of memories of dreams provoked by waking subjects during paradoxical sleep (*dream recall*), was for long the only testimony of dreaming. It has remained the battlefield of psychologists and psychiatrists on which the diverse psychoanalytical schools confront each other. More pragmatically, experimental neurophysiology has devoted itself to the analysis of neurobiological mechanisms of paradoxical sleep in animals.

### The Mechanisms That Prepare Dreams

As we learned in chapter 1, there is an arousal system formed by a network of neurons in the reticular formation of the midbrain (see figure 1) that is responsible for the waking state. During arousal these neurons excite the cerebral cortex using their neurotransmitters, especially acetylcholine. They themselves receive an innervation, notably from the locus ceruleus, a tiny group of neurons in the pons (see figure 1). This innervation uses norepinephrine as transmitter (figure 7).

Under normal circumstances, paradoxical sleep never appears during waking. Direct transition from waking to paradoxical sleep is only seen during narcolepsy (see above). It must always be initiated by a preliminary phase of slow wave sleep. The mechanisms of this preparatory phase are complex, but we understand their major principles. First of all, the waking state must end, so the brain's arousal system must not be excited. This supposes that there is no immediate personal danger, and that this is being signaled by a lack of auditory, visual, and olfactory inputs from potential predators, and that no pain receptors are being excited. It also supposes that the needs of the organism are satisfied (the animal is neither hungry nor thirsty, it is at the right temperature, is not searching for a sexual partner, and so on). Finally, it supposes also that the period of sleep is during a daily (circadian) phase of inactivity; for instance, we know that sleep comes spontaneously to the rat more easily in the daytime than at night. If all these conditions are fulfilled, the arousal system is no longer excited and *active* mechanisms for falling asleep are triggered.

Falling asleep involves other structures in the brainstem, and in particular part of the *raphe* system (see figure 7). These are small-celled nuclei close to the midline of the reticular formation, and their neurons contain serotonin.

So now we have a brain system to explain sleep itself. But why did evolution invent dreaming, at least in warm-blooded animals?

A possible beginning of an explanation is again offered by the reductionist approach of experimental neurophysiology which over thirty years ago succeeded in dissecting the intrinsic machinery of dreaming and answering the following questions (figure 7). What brain structures are necessary and adequate for the periodic triggering of the phenomena of dreams? How do they interact? And where are the systems that prevent dreams from occurring during waking rather than after a fairly long period of sleep?

## Paradoxical Sleep

We have now seen several times that dreams appear at the same time as an ensemble of specific physiological activities that we call paradoxical sleep. This phase of sleep is paradoxical in that intense cerebral activity coincides with muscle atonia.

We can recognize slow wave sleep from paradoxical sleep and from waking thanks to recordings of activity through electrodes implanted in the brain and muscles in nonanesthetized, freely moving animals (figure 8). During paradoxical sleep we can identify *tonic* (persistent) signs and *phasic* (episodic) signs. Tonic signs are, for instance, cortical activation similar to that of the wide-awake state and generalized muscle relaxation. Phasic signs include a very special electrical activity of the brain that was first described in the *pons*, the lateral *geniculate* nucleus, and the *occipital* cortex (see figure 8). This led to the term *ponto-geniculo-occipital* (PGO) activity. It is responsible for the peripheral phasic phenomena of dreaming such as rapid eye movements, movements of the whiskers of a cat, its tongue, sometimes its toes, and more rarely its tail. During paradoxical sleep, of course, the absence of postural tone means that there are only very rarely coordinated movements of limb muscles. A dog may have generalized movements of its four limbs and even sometimes growl or bark. However, no matter how brisk these movements, they will never lead to the animal getting up or walking.

When paradoxical sleep was identified at the end of the 1950s the situation was as follows. All the evidence pointed to human dreaming occurring during REM sleep, but a similar sleep state existed in cats, and in other mammals. So why refuse to recognize the faculty of dreaming in cats simply because cats

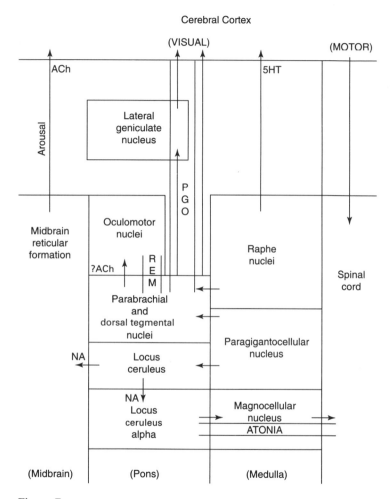

**Figure 7**
Schematic drawing of the structures involved in the three states of brain function. The cerebral cortex is at the top of the figure and the brainstem (midbrain, pons, and medulla) at the bottom. During *waking* there is activation of aminergic systems: serotoninergic (5HT) from the raphe nuclei and noradrenergic (NA) from the locus ceruleus. The raphe excites the cortex directly, while the locus ceruleus excites

could not relate them to us? Now, obviously it is impossible for a cat to describe its dreams, but can we extend our analysis of the phenomena that take place during paradoxical sleep? The problem for the neurophysiologist is as follows: are REMs just an epiphenomenon reflecting anarchic activation of motor neurons, or are they part of a structured, integrated motor behavior that is trapped somewhere in the central nervous system? If so, is it possible to untrap the motor program and externalize the behavior of a dreaming cat, its *oneiric behavior*? Before replying positively to this question, we must describe a few more details of the organization of the structures and mechanisms that take part in the setting up and maintenance of paradoxical sleep.

## What Parts of the Brain Are Needed to Trigger Dreaming?

Ablation of the cerebral cortex does not affect the onset of paradoxical sleep significantly. What is more, in spite of complete ablation of structures in front of the pons, including the hypothalamus and the pituitary gland (see figure 1), paradoxical sleep continues to appear periodically. Its characteristic electrical signals appear in the pons, accompanying eye movements and changes in heart rate and breathing. So, as the pons

the midbrain reticular formation which excites the cortex with acetylcholine (ACh). *Slow wave (light) sleep* is maintained by these same systems. The locus ceruleus also inhibits the locus ceruleus alpha. This inhibition ceases with the onset of *paradoxical (REM) sleep*. Then the PGO system begins at the parabrachial and dorsal tegmental nuclei of the *p*ons, is transmitted to the lateral geniculate nucleus, and finally to the visual cortex of the occipital lobe. At the same time the locus ceruleus alpha excites the magnocellular nucleus of the medulla, which then sends messages down the reticulospinal tract to inhibit motor activity in the spinal cord.

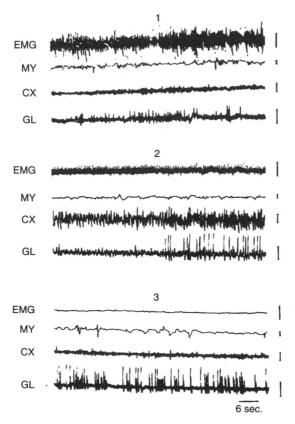

**Figure 8**
The main criteria used to recognize waking (1), slow wave sleep (2), and paradoxical sleep (3) in the cat. The signs of paradoxical sleep are resumption of cortical activity (CX), recorded here in the visual cortex, like that in waking, and complete postural atonia (EMG). The particular activity recorded in certain parts of the brain, such as the pons, the lateral geniculate nucleus (GL), and the occipital cortex (PGO activity), is one of the major keys to an explanation of paradoxical sleep. It is the central phenomenon responsible for, among other things, the characteristic rapid eye movements (MY) of paradoxical sleep.

and the medulla alone are adequate for paradoxical sleep to appear periodically, they must contain "executive" systems for it.

It is as if numerous control mechanisms prevent the start of paradoxical sleep during waking and in the early phases of sleep. The two most important are situated in a part of the arousal system (the locus ceruleus) and in the raphe group (which is active during waking, falling asleep, and light sleep). Paradoxical sleep can only appear when all activity in these structures has ceased.

So we see that dreaming is only possible after checking several safety systems: this protection seems very appropriate, for dreaming is accompanied by a considerable increase in the arousal threshold and almost complete paralysis. Deaf, blind, and paralyzed, the individual becomes very vulnerable. He can only dream if he is in security, for only then can he plunge safely into deep sleep. This concept of security is important and partly explains variations in the duration of dreams in different species. Hunted animals, rarely secure, sleep little and very lightly, and the total duration of periods of paradoxical sleep does not exceed 15 to 20 minutes per 24 hours. On the other hand, hunters (carnivores), including the domestic cat who lives in perfect safety and does not need to hunt for food, sleep a lot and their paradoxical sleep can last more than 200 minutes per 24 hours.

### Brainstem "Executive" Structures for Paradoxical Sleep: The Machinery of Dreaming

As we have said, the main external signs of paradoxical sleep are postural atonia and rapid eye movements, whereas the internal signs are cortical and PGO activity. Which brain structures trigger them? We saw just now that they must be in the brainstem (see figure 1), but their precise identification has been long and difficult in view of the complex organization of the brainstem reticular formation. However, this research has made regular progress thanks to new anatomical and histochemical techniques.

### Postural Atonia

Postural atonia can be triggered by exciting various systems; remember that in man cataplexy can be provoked by laughing! During paradoxical sleep we can record increased activity of neurons in many structures, but often this activity is related to associated phenomena such as eye movements. However, we have narrowed down the location of the command system for postural atonia thanks to studies of the effects of localized brainstem lesions, but particularly to microelectrode recordings made by Kasuya Sakai and his colleagues[136,137] at the Faculty of Medicine in Lyon. What we know can be summarized as follows. It looks complicated at first sight, but is quite logical if followed step by step and related to figures 1 and 7.

Postural atonia during paradoxical sleep is caused by inhibitory motor activity at three levels. Let us liken this activity to a brake. The first level is a command level and the others are executive levels. The command level is in a small group of neurons, situated alongside the locus ceruleus, called the *locus ceruleus alpha*. These neurons are sensitive to acetylcholine, for they can be stimulated by localized injection of carbachol, a drug that mimics acetylcholine. Carbachol produces generalized atonia either during paradoxical sleep or during waking (cataplexy). This nucleus is normally inhibited during waking and normal sleep by the locus ceruleus itself, whose neurons release norepinephrine.

Thus, during waking and sleeping the electrical activity of the *locus ceruleus is high*, while that of the *locus ceruleus alpha is zero*. The activity of the locus ceruleus diminishes gradually during slow wave sleep, then stops completely at the start of paradoxical sleep, allowing excitation of the locus ceruleus alpha. The locus ceruleus alpha begins to be active a few minutes before paradoxical sleep, reaching maximum discharge rates during a dream and stopping completely at its end.[84]

Excitatory signals are then sent to the second level, in the medulla, along a descending pontomedullary pathway. When they arrive at the *magnocellular nucleus* of the reticular formation (so called because it contains large cells) they excite it. The magnocellular nucleus corresponds to the "inhibitory reticular formation" discovered by Horace Magoun and Ruth Rhines.[103] Its neurons therefore also increase in activity during paradoxical sleep.

Then it sends descending inhibitory signals along the *reticulospinal* tract to the spinal cord. There, at the motor neurons that innervate the muscles directly, they block excitation coming from the motor area of the cerebral cortex (itself excited by PGO activity) and produce postural atonia.[22] Sometimes a few motor signals cross this inhibitory barrier, causing small movements of the fingers, or the ears and whiskers (in cats), but essentially only the eye and respiratory muscles escape this intense inhibitory activity.

It is unlikely that other brainstem structures contribute to the control of postural atonia. Extensive lesions made by tiny injections of a neurotoxic agent that selectively destroys nerve cell bodies without destroying their axons (the nerve fibers that conduct information from the cell body toward other cells) in other parts of the pontine reticular formation have no effect on paradoxical sleep. For instance, almost total destruction of the *gigantocellular* nucleus of the reticular formation, which contains giant neurons sending axons forward in the brain or back toward the spinal cord, has no effect on paradoxical sleep. This is all the more astonishing in that electrical activity in this gigantocellular nucleus increases considerably during paradoxical sleep (and waking), and certain people have considered it as the real executive system of paradoxical sleep. It also seems that this nucleus is not related to controlling eye movements during dreaming. So what does it do? Another unfathomed mystery of dreaming.

### The Ponto-Geniculo-Occipital System

The PGO system, which we discussed briefly above, is more complex than the one that is responsible for postural atonia.[136,137,151] However, its study has been facilitated by the fact that it can be excited by drugs or lesions whose common denominator is suppression of the liberation of serotonin from the raphe nuclei. One can use reserpine, parachlorophenylalanine, or even destroy parts of the raphe nuclei. These different techniques all lead to the appearance of continuous PGO activity during waking.

The PGO system is composed of "generators" and of various pathways (see figure 7). The topography of the neurons (very probably cholinergic) that constitute the PGO generators has been worked out in detail. They are in the pontine reticular formation (the *parabrachial* and the *dorsal tegmental* nuclei). The generators are like automatic pacemakers, for periodic PGO activity can still be recorded from the pons in an animal with the pons isolated from the rest of the brain.[75,106]

The system that conducts PGO information from the pons to the lateral geniculate nucleus and to visual cortical areas has been identified. From each generator a pathway ascends to terminate either at the lateral geniculate nucleus or the visual cortex.[96] The pontine generator also sends excitatory signals to the oculomotor nuclei that are responsible for eye movements during paradoxical sleep.[20]

So we can define the primary PGO system anatomically and observe its activity in the form of the slow, high-amplitude waves that characterize paradoxical sleep. However, the PGO generators are not limited to exciting just the visual and oculomotor systems. With microelectrodes it is possible to detect traces of their activity in the great majority of neurons in the reticular formation, the thalamus, and the cerebral cortex (especially its interneurons, the intrinsic cells whose axons excite or inhibit other cortical neurons), as demonstrated by Mircea Steriade from Laval University in Quebec.[148,150] Among others, they influence neurons of the motor systems responsible for voluntary and postural motor activity. Indeed, if we place a microelectrode anywhere in the brain there is about a 60% chance of recording a neuron that is influenced (either excited or inhibited) by activity in the PGO generator.

Excitatory motor activity reaches the spinal cord, which during waking would set off gestures and behavioral patterns. But normally during paradoxical sleep the brake system commanded by the locus ceruleus alpha takes over to inhibit this motor activity, blocking the motor neurons of the cord by means of a powerful descending inhibition, as described above.

### Permissive Systems
The concept of a "permissive" system has emerged recently in the literature. It is rather confusing but has, alas, become widespread. It means that inactivation of such systems permits dreams to occur. The terms "inhibitory" or "blocking" systems might be preferable.

These systems include the serotoninergic neurons in the raphe system and the noradrenergic neurons in the locus ceruleus (see figure 7), as well as histamine-containing neurons in the hypothalamus. As we saw above, they are active during waking. So, waking leads to sleeping, as in Zarathustra's adage: *No small art is it to sleep: it is necessary for that purpose to keep awake all day.* We do not yet know the exact cause of the decreased activity in such aminergic systems at the beginning of paradoxical sleep, and during it. It probably depends on many factors. However, it seems that a group of cells in the medulla (in the region called the *paragigantocellular* area) may play an important role. These cells are responsible for control of the sympathetic nervous system, which regulates such basic functions as heart rate, blood pressure, and respiration, and seem to be the principal neurons that excite the locus ceruleus. Reduced activity in sympathetic excitatory neurons causes a peripheral vasodilation during sleep, leading to loss of heat and therefore lowered body temperature. It is possible that it also causes loss of excitation in permissive systems. Thus we can speculate objectively about a relationship between temperature control and sleeping and dreaming. Such a relationship is not easy to analyze. Does the sleep-wake cycle control body temperature cycles? Or is it the converse? Was paradoxical sleep a consequence of the invention of warm-bloodedness by a common ancestor of birds and mammals, or an independent invention during their long evolutionary history?

## Periodicity in Dreaming

A major problem for neurophysiology to solve concerns the significance of periodicity in dreaming. Why does the dream machine function periodically rather than continuously?

The ultradian (occurring several times a day) periodicity of dreams during sleep is a characteristic of a species.[121] It is fairly closely related to the logarithm of its body weight, and thus to its metabolism. For a rat it is 10 minutes, in cats it is 25 minutes, in man 90 minutes, and in elephants 180 minutes (see figure 6). In addition, the average duration of each episode of dreaming is also correlated with species: two minutes for the rat, five for the cat, and twenty for humans.[107]

So, the periodic generator for dreams during sleep obeys a relatively simple law. In most species, dreams occupy about a quarter of its sleep (six per twenty-five minutes in cats, twenty per ninety minutes in man). Experiments in our laboratory have shown that it is possible to vary either the duration or the periodicity in animals by modifying brain metabolism by changing either the temperature (energy demand) or the oxygen supply (energy supply). The periodicity of dreams seems then to be controlled by central *economic* factors (the relationship between energy supply and demand). One could explain this relationship metaphorically: dreams seem to imply a large expenditure of energy (increased glucose, and probably oxygen, consumption), whereas arousal needs increased glucose *without* increased oxygen.

One of the functions of sleep could be to prepare the necessary energy conditions for dreams: decreased body temperature (i.e., reduced energy demand), decreased oxygen consumption, and deposit of energy reserves as glycogen stored in the cells which "feed" the neurons, that is, the glial cells.[57,89] *When, and only when*, enough energy reserves have been accumulated, a dream can take place and use those reserves, probably through a different metabolic pathway from that of the waking state.

It thus seems that dream consciousness uses more energy than waking consciousness. That is why any factors that increase brain energy requirements (such as overheating or fever or decreased energy supply through hypoxia or ischemia) suppress dreaming but can increase wakefulness or sleep.

The need to renew energy reserves during slow wave sleep explains, at least partially, why systems responsible for dreaming can only work periodically.

## Sleep as the Guardian of Paradoxical Sleep, and the Condition for its Appearance

To go to sleep signifies for an animal that certain eco-ethological conditions have been met: absence of external (predators) or internal (pain) danger, that is, an absence of triggering of arousal systems. Thus there is a significant relationship between the amount of paradoxical sleep (and therefore of total sleep) and security factors.[5] Sleep is thus the guardian of paradoxical sleep, a potentially dangerous situation for the survival of the individual because of the increased threshold for arousal and the paralysis of its principal muscles.

The appearance of slow wave sleep in the circadian cycle also signifies that environmental conditions are close to thermal neutrality (27 °C). Basal metabolism is therefore low, and the processes implicated in slow wave sleep will progressively lower the brain's temperature and its consumption of glucose and oxygen, while energy reserves accumulate as glycogen in glial cells.[57, 89] At the same time the activity of arousal systems (such as catecholaminergic, serotoninergic, and histaminergic systems) diminishes, preparing the conditions necessary for paradoxical sleep, some of which seem to stimulate energy cycles.

Paradoxical sleep is, indeed, accompanied by a consumption of glucose at least equal to that during waking, as has been revealed by deoxyglucose experiments in animals or PET scanning in humans, both of which depend on visualizing local metabolic changes in the brain using radioactively labeled glucose or other chemicals.[51,128] It is probable, although not yet proved, that there is also increased consumption of oxygen. Paradoxical sleep is indeed *selectively* suppressed by hypoxia (which can increase slow wave sleep or arousal).[7] The utilization of glucose depends on the aerobic (Krebs) cycle. This cycle is necessary for the synthesis of acetylcholine[56] regulated by pyruvate dehydrogenase (PDH). This enzyme can be periodically activated or inactivated by the level of the redox potential or by the intermediary of hormones, such as prolactin or insulin.[155] PDH could then play an important, but probably not exclusive, role in determining the periodicity of paradoxical sleep. It is interesting to note that cholinergic neurons in the pons and medulla (some of which are responsible for paradoxical sleep) are particularly rich in PDH.[111]

In conclusion, slow wave sleep prepares conditions suitable for the appearance of paradoxical sleep in several ways. Its appearance is indicative of both absence of excitation in waking systems and an ambient temperature close to neutral, allowing decreased metabolic and sympathetic activity and brain temperature, as well as the filling of energy reserves. These processes seem necessary for the activation of brainstem cholinergic neurons, responsible for paradoxical sleep, via the oxidative pyruvate pathway. Thus paradoxical sleep seems dependent on the neurotransmitter acetylcholine, the synthesis of which seems closely controlled by energy factors.

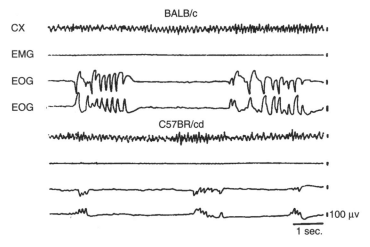

**Figure 9**
Eye movements (EOG) during paradoxical sleep are different in different strains of mice. Crossing the mice, and backcrosses of the progeniture with the parents, permits the demonstration of the existence of a genetic factor in the organization of eye movements. CX, cortical activity; EMG, electromyogram. (From Cespuglio et al.[21])

## Are Dreams in Our Genes?

I believe that PGO activity is the key to the mystery of dreaming. Is PGO activity related to previously experienced events, or is it independent of a person's life? The beginnings of an answer are provided by genetics in the only animal capable of dreaming on which genetic experiments can be conducted, because of its many well-studied strains: the mouse. It seems that the message delivered by the dream generator is subject to genetic determination, each strain of mouse having a different sleep pattern (figure 9).[21] More recently, experiments on identical human twins have shown the similarity of the pattern of their eye movements compared with nonidentical twins. So it seems as if the genetic makeup of each individual may be expressed in dreams.

We are getting to the heart of the problem—the battlefield of ideological quarrels—nature versus nurture. The question is as follows. If dreaming turns out to be due to genetically controlled programming of the brain, might it be responsible for individual variation in instinctive behavior in animals, and for the hereditary part of our human personality? That is the part that is little, if at all, influenced by environment, culture, or learning—our "psychological heredity."

Since Locke, environmentalists have said *Homo fit non nascitur*. *Homo nascitur non fit* have replied the nativists in support of innate ability. It would be better to reply, as did Shakespeare, "We are such stuff as dreams are made on."

## The Phylogeny of Dreams

Is dreaming (or paradoxical sleep) an attribute of all animals, at least of all vertebrates? (dreams are difficult to recognize in a bacterium, an oyster, or a mosquito). The answer is no: no one has yet been able to record unequivocally a state similar to paradoxical sleep in fish, amphibians, or reptiles (except perhaps in the crocodile), whereas it is relatively easy to demonstrate alternating sleep-wake cycles in fish and amphibians and variations in the electrical activity of the brain during sleep in reptiles. It looks as if lower (cold-blooded) vertebrates have never "needed" paradoxical sleep.

In contrast, it is easy to demonstrate paradoxical sleep in birds and mammals, the warm-blooded animals. Their ultradian rhythm is closely correlated with brain metabolism and weight. Paradoxical sleep exists in birds for very short periods (five to fifteen seconds) and it only accounts for 3% to 5% of the total duration of sleep. There are considerable variations among species, from chickens (which only dream for twenty-five minutes each night, like cows) to chimpanzees (ninety minutes) to man (100 minutes). The champion dreamer is the domestic cat (200 minutes per day). A notable exception is the dolphin in which paradoxical sleep has not been demonstrated.[113] So brain complexity is not a criterion on which to measure the amount of dreaming in a given species. This is why many other correlations have been proposed. One of the best is an index of *security*. Animals that are secure in their natural surroundings sleep more easily than those in danger of attack, and sleep will be more readily accompanied by dreams.

The phylogeny of dreaming thus leaves us with an unsolved enigma, all the more difficult to explain when one considers the mystery of the dolphin. So let us consider our marine cousin, endowed as it is with great brain power. First of all it is subject to Ondine's curse, for it must breathe voluntarily, so it must choose between staying awake or drowning! The idea of security is very much involved here! Evolution has resolved this choice very elegantly, for the dolphin sleeps with one side of its brain at a time, controlling its respiration alternately with the left or right hemisphere (figure 10). In spite of many years of research led by my friend Lev Mukhametov in Moscow and in the Crimea, it has so far proved impossible to record periods of paradoxical sleep in dolphins.[113] This absence of proof is not a proof of absence, but while this enigma remains unresolved, any theory of the functions of dreams must remain tentative.

The passage from cold- to warm-bloodedness was also accompanied by changes in the brain (the appearance of "cortical" structures such as the archistriatum in birds and the

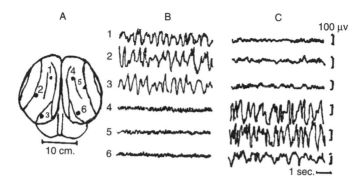

**Figure 10**
The dolphin only sleeps with one hemisphere at a time. (A) Drawing
of the positions of electrodes on the cerebral cortex of a dolphin. (B)
Slow wave sleep in the right hemisphere, while the left hemisphere is
awake (rapid activity). (C) Twenty minutes later the left hemisphere is
asleep, whereas the right is active. (From Mukhametov et al.[114])

cerebral cortex in mammals), as well as in the whole organism
(a considerable increase in energy handling, enabling a change
from slow metabolism to fast metabolism). Another very important phenomenon affected the brain. Whereas neurogenesis
(the birth of new neurons by cell division) persists throughout
the life of cold-blooded animals, this capacity is lost in warm-
blooded ones.[157] It can persist in some birds, and may be
responsible for the genetic transmission of the canary's
song.[122] Neurogenesis stops during the first weeks of life in the
rat and the kitten, or halfway through gestation in the human
fetus.

## The Ontogeny of Dreams

The first postnatal days of a rat or kitten are marked by the
alternation of two states. The first is adaptive waking behavior

of the still cold-blooded neonate during which it instinctively seeks food and warmth in its mother's fur. This alternates with an immature form of paradoxical sleep, or *active* sleep, as we saw in chapter 1. Polygraph recordings from guinea pig fetuses in utero, or during the first two weeks after birth in rats and kittens, have enabled us to describe this state more fully. The animal's eyes, ears, paws, and tail move spasmodically in an incessant bout of motor neuronal activity. There is no electrophysiological sign of paradoxical sleep, such as variations in cortical activity and PGO activity, and electroshock, drugs, and lesions that suppress paradoxical sleep in adults do not affect active sleep.[1] It is almost continuous during the first few days and has no obvious periodicity.[87,152] It is thus very probable that active sleep involves spontaneous movements, observed in many embryos, accompanying neurogenesis at the end of cerebral maturation.[26,61]

Little by little, as genetic programming and neurogenesis in the nervous system come to an end, brainstem structures and PGO systems become organized so that true paradoxical sleep replaces active sleep and occupies a major part (40%) of sleep. Typical polygraphic signs of paradoxical sleep (cortical activity, PGO activity, and atonia) only appear toward the end of the second week. It becomes more and more like that of adults and after twenty-one days all the major features are visible, including obvious periodicity. The muscle twitches disappear, leaving only rapid eye movements. From this time it is possible to increase or suppress paradoxical sleep with the same drugs as in the adult.

The nature of active sleep during the first few postnatal days is still debated. Is it already a primitive form of paradoxical sleep? Or does it represent the end of an "embryonic" state?

The second explanation seems the more plausible, for active sleep accompanies the end of neurogenesis. PGO activity, which helps trigger paradoxical sleep, does not appear until the third week of life in the kitten.[3] In addition, it is unlikely that the muscle twitches of active sleep reflect activity in the brainstem generator of paradoxical sleep. Indeed, Adrien observed that in rats twitches of the hind limbs are not suppressed by total section of the spinal cord. What is more, it is almost impossible to suppress active sleep in rats and kittens during the first postnatal week by electroshock, although it does suppress paradoxical sleep after the second week. But above all, lesions in specific brainstem nuclei do not suppress active sleep during the first two weeks, whereas such operations suppress paradoxical sleep, as in the adult, after the third week.[1,26]

Many studies have established that the more immature the newborn mammal (and the more fragile its thermoregulation), the more active sleep it has: 50% to 60% of sleeping time for a human neonate, 80% to 90% for a kitten or rat. It has even been demonstrated that the fetus of a guinea pig in utero has a considerably greater amount of active sleep than the adult (figure 11). The same is true of the chick embryo in ovo a few days before hatching, a marsupial in the pouch, and a premature human baby in incubatione, all of which demonstrate major polygraphic features of paradoxical sleep during their active sleep. Their eye movements cannot be related to possible dream images, for the visual pathways and the cortex are not yet fully developed. Neurophysiological mechanisms are thus already in place before the appearance of dream consciousness, just as they precede consciousness itself.

Thus it is at the moment that the maturation and genetic programming of neurons are ending that active sleep, which

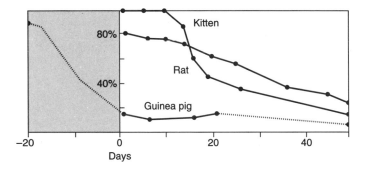

**Figure 11**
On the ordinate, the percentage of immative paradoxical (active) sleep compared with the total duration of sleep in the kitten, the rat pup, and the guinea pig. The guinea pig is born with an almost mature nervous system and its quantity of active sleep is low, as in most herbivores. In contrast, the guinea pig fetus manifests a high proportion of active sleep twenty days before birth when the maturation of its brain is similar to that of newborn cats and rats. Days before and after birth are on the abscissa. (From Jouvet-Mounier et al.[87])

will later become the true paradoxical sleep of dreaming, reaches its maximum, and declines from then on. You must admit that this is a very strange phenomenon.

# 3

## Dream Memories

The first studies of paradoxical sleep were mainly due to an interest in dreams. Do we really dream during paradoxical sleep, and is paradoxical sleep the only time when dreams can appear?

The periods of REM sleep in humans were initially considered as light sleep (see figures 3 and 4). The equating of REM sleep with paradoxical sleep, considered as a *state* in its own right, deeper than the deepest sleep, was not an easy transition to make. Even after the concept of it as a state had won the day, a few decades were necessary to convince the worst skeptics that dreaming was not a continuous process during sleep but that it depended totally on the periodic appearance of paradoxical sleep.[30]

At first many people were still influenced by the work of Maury (for whom dreaming was a half-awake state) and Freud (for whom the dream was the guardian of sleep), and found it difficult to imagine that paradoxical sleep or REM sleep was a period of deep sleep, let alone a new state as such. How could a

From an article published in *La Revue du Praticien* (1979) 1: 29–32. Part of it formed the basis for a lecture presented at the meeting of the Association for Psychophysiological Study of Sleep in Palo Alto, California in 1978.

state of deep sleep be the guardian of sleep, for a guardian must be vigilant? Now, the concept of dreaming as a third state is almost universally recognized. Nevertheless, we still find in some sleep laboratories that paradoxical or REM sleep is classed as light sleep (stage 1) on hypnograms (records made during sleep) (see figures 3 and 4). Developments between 1953 and 1986 demonstrated the close relationship in humans between paradoxical or REM sleep and dreaming as long as the definitions were clear.

## The Three Paths to Dreams

As we have seen so far, study of the mechanisms and function (or functions) of dreaming has followed three main paths. The first explores dreaming from the "inside," studying the subjective content of dreams by analyzing recalled memories of them. The other two are objective and experimental, exploring dreams from the "outside"; they depend on the hypothesis that the mechanisms of dreaming are the same as those of paradoxical sleep, its neurobiological basis.

## The Approach from the "Outside"

One of these approaches is frankly reductionist. Experimental neurophysiology has enabled us to identify systems of neurons in the brainstem that fire synchronously and cause paradoxical sleep (see chapter 2).

The other experimental method has a more global, holistic approach, describing the natural history of paradoxical sleep in terms of phylogenetic and ontogenetic evolution. Study of the natural history of paradoxical sleep, like the reductionist approach even pushed to its furthest molecular extremes, does not enable us to explain the *functions* of paradoxical sleep. They will perhaps one day be explained when we understand the functions of their component parts better, but they cannot immediately be deduced from them.

## The Approach from the "Inside": The Study of Dream Recall

The first and oldest approach is that of the study of what we remember of our dreams. Does it also lead to a dead end?

Experimental neurophysiology can help in a limited way. In the cat it is possible to destroy selectively the system responsible for the inhibition of muscle tone during paradoxical sleep, which we examined in chapter 2. After such a lesion animals demonstrate stereotyped behavior during each period of paradoxical sleep: visual exploration, stalking, pursuit, capture, rage, or fear. This is *oneiric behavior*,[79] and we shall come back to it in more detail in chapter 4. But how can we know if our cat is dreaming of a bird, a mouse, or a predator?

So the neurophysiologist is obliged to study recalled memories of dreams in the *human being*. This approach is strewn with pitfalls. Is a recalled dream the exact reflection of the oneiric scene, or is it immediately corrupted by waking consciousness? What is more, as the object of the study is the subject of a dream, it is all too easy to inadvertently modify our interpretation of our own memories.

In spite of these reservations, an exploration of the contents of a long series of recalled dreams might enable us to reveal significant features susceptible to a neurobiological interpretation and to the formulation of hypotheses. These would obviously have to await proof or refutation in the light of further series of recalled dreams: one day "dream banks" may be set up.

In 1981 Dement[35] summarized eight worldwide studies of dream recall when waking subjects during slow wave or REM sleep: "... we were able to report on a total of 214 subjects, both male and female, studied on 885 subject-nights of sleep. Sleep was interrupted 2,240 times during the REM phase, and these awakenings elicited 1,864 instances of 'vivid dream recall,' a recall rate of 83.3 percent. When compared to the overall (non-REM) results, the REM period was unquestionably established as the time when the probability of being able to recall a dream is maximal."

However, the researchers noticed subsequently that they had neglected to determine precisely what would or would not be defined as a dream, and to decide on a mutual definition. In other words, "What is a dream?"

It was David Foulkes[48] who highlighted the absolute necessity for precise definition by a study of dream recall after waking during slow wave sleep. Dement[35] described events around that time: "He counted as dream recall any report of mental content, including what might be called 'thinking' reports. Subjects, when awakened, were asked, 'Was anything going through your mind?' rather than, 'Were you dreaming?' Foulkes' approach almost certainly elicited the reporting of additional material that was not specifically labeled as dreaming by the subjects. As a consequence, Foulkes obtained a much higher percentage of 'dream recall' from (non-REM) sleep than any previous investigator."

How can we differentiate the "dream" reports from the "thinking" reports? A graduate student of Allan Rechtschaffen, Gene Orlinsky, devised an eight-point scale for judging dream reports:

0. Subject cannot remember dreaming; no dream is reported upon awakening.

1. Subject remembers having dreamed, or thinks he may have dreamed, but cannot remember any specific content.

2. Subject remembers a specific topic, but in isolation; for example, a fragmentary action, scene, object, word, or idea unrelated to anything else.

3. Subject remembers several disconnected thoughts, scenes or actions.

4. Subject remembers a short but coherent dream, the parts of which seem related to each other; for example, a conversation rather than a word, a problem worked through rather than an idea, a purposeful rather than a fragmentary action.

5. Subject remembers a detailed dream sequence in which something happens followed by some consequence, or in which one scene, mood, or main interacting character is replaced by another (different from 3 either in coherence or change in the development of the several parts of the sequence).

6. Subject remembers a long, detailed dream sequence involving three or four discernible stages of development.

7. Subject remembers an extremely long and detailed dream sequence of five or more stages; or more than one dream (at least one of which is rated 5) for a single awakening."[35]

Of 400 replies after waking during slow wave sleep, Orlinsky discovered that 57% fell into classes 1 to 7. When he looked only at classes 2 to 7 the percentage fell to 46% and it fell further as he excluded one lower class after another. Only 7% fell into classes 6 and 7. So this study underlined clearly that the proportion of dreams during slow wave sleep depends essentially on the criteria utilized to define dream recall. This explains the variations found in different studies on slow wave sleep.

Subsequent researchers have tried to compare typical recall during slow wave and paradoxical sleep. Dement[35] quotes the following examples from an article by Rechtschaffen and his colleagues.[132]

Report from a subject woken during slow wave sleep: "I had been dreaming about getting ready to take some kind of an exam. It had been a very short dream. That's just about all that it contained. I don't think I was worried about it."

Report from the same subject woken during REM sleep later the same night: "I was dreaming about exams. In the early part of the dream, I was dreaming that I had just finished taking an exam and it was a very sunny day outside. I was walking with a boy who was in some of my classes with me. There was a sort of a ... a break, and someone mentioned a grade they had gotten in a social science exam, and I asked them if the social science marks had come in. They said yes. I didn't get mine because I had been away for a day."[132]

Dement pointed out that, in spite of the continuity of theme, the second report obviously contained much more of the perceptual vividness and organization usually associated with dreams. Compared with periods of paradoxical sleep, mental activity during slow wave sleep is generally more poorly recalled. It is closer to *thinking* than *dreaming*, less vivid, less visual, more conceptual, subject to greater voluntary control, more related to everyday life, and it occurs during lighter sleep. The content is less emotional, even pleasant.

In the light of these studies we conclude that dreams reach the height of their development and structure during paradoxical sleep. We could imagine that slow wave sleep prepares the outline of a dream, still at this stage in the form of thoughts and reflections without the contribution of all the sensory and motor faculties. Then, during paradoxical sleep, the final form of the dream blossoms in all its sensory splendor, with vision, sound, smell, and taste, and its varied emotional and motor trappings.

The material I shall now describe comprises 2525 memories I recorded immediately after a dream during the night, or on waking in the morning, between December 1970 and August 1978, making an average of 0.9 memories per night! The maximum was nine in a night, and the longest period without dream recall was nine days. A preliminary, very incomplete study of this material already reveals features related to recent memory, and others pointing to separate activity in the two cerebral hemispheres.

**Dreams and Recent Memory**

If we eliminate recalled dreams relating to events more than fifteen days earlier, we have a collection of 400 in which we can date an event occurring in the dream precisely to between 0 and 14 days. Of these, 130 were experienced during normal daily life, and 270 during or just after foreign travel.

Figure 12 shows the distribution of latencies between an event and its dream recall. Events from the same day (*day residues*, with 0 latency) occurred 45 times out of 130 (35%). This high occurrence rate confirms a classic subjective concept. Thereafter there was a rapid tailing off to the sixth day. This diminution was, however, interrupted by a significant peak of dreams about events eight days earlier (13 out of 130, or 10%).

The recollection of events eight days previously was mainly found when studying dreams during journeys or in the fifteen days following them. Analysis of twenty journeys (five to twenty days long) revealed a latency of seven or eight days for the incorporation of scenes from a journey into oneiric space. So, of 104 dreams recalled during the first six days of a journey, only one contained a scene from the new environment, even when the journey involved an exotic location, or a sea

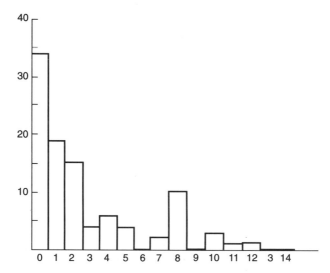

**Figure 12**
Histogram of the distribution of latencies between events and their incorporation in 130 dreams. On the ordinate are the percentages. On the abscissa are the latencies. 0 indicates same-day memories (day residues), 1 indicates events of the previous day, and so on. There is a significant peak at 8 days.

cruise. Recollections from the same day involving the dreamer or other persons were either set in an unknown location or an environment familiar before the journey. From the seventh day there was an increasing number of recalled dreams incorporating scenery influenced by the new location. This latency was found again on returning from a journey, for dream recall involving the place visited continued each night for seven or eight days (figure 13).

The following hypothesis would explain the significant peak of eight-day-old memories involving everyday life, and the seven- or eight-day latency needed for the incorporation of a new scene in a dream. We may assume that the process

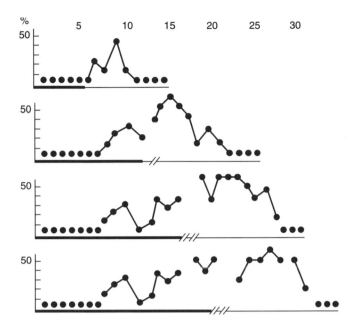

**Figure 13**
Appearance of spatial memory during dreams. On the ordinate: percentage of dreams associated with a visit to a foreign country. On
the abscissa: the heavy horizontal line indicates journeys of different
durations (5, 10, 15, or 20 days). Note the appearance of dream recall
associated with the journey on about the seventh or eighth day and the
persistence of dream recall after the end of the journey and the return
home. The short oblique lines indicate a total absence of dream recall
due to the actual return journey.

of dreaming uses two sorts of memory. The first is devoid of
spatial content and relates to very recent events. This memory,
responsible for recollections from the same day, diminishes
rapidly over six or seven days. The second type of memory is
spatial, remains latent in the dream scene for six or seven days,
and is responsible for memories of the environment.

In the more usual case of life in a familiar and stable environment, it is difficult to recall a specific piece of scenery in the dream theater, for most scenes take place in familiar places (the workplace, home, or a daily journey). The chances of same-day memories being related to a familiar scene are very high. This does not permit us to conclude that a familiar scene is always part of same-day memories. What is more, a familiar environment may not contain enough specific elements to enable us to put a precise date on memories of events eight days earlier. On the other hand, during journeys, the novelty and diversity of the environment enable us to date fairly precisely the location of the dream scene, and to easily distinguish ephemeral, spaceless memories from the spatial memories that only appear after a latency of eight days.

This latency of spatial memory appears in various anecdotes. At the beginning of their detention, prisoners' dreams take place in locations associated with their previous life of freedom, whereas after leaving prison their dreams continue to take place in their cell.

These data only concern recent memories. It is probable that an exhaustive analysis of all my 2525 dream memories would reveal other features of their pattern of recurrence in relation to more distant events, regardless of whether they had been incorporated in previous dream memories.

It is still too early to suggest a neurobiological basis for latency in the reutilization of our environment in our dreams. If this phenomenon is confirmed in other series of recalled dreams it would suggest that there might exist specific circuits or mechanisms for memorizing our environment. This information could be used without latency during waking, but would be subject to temporary deletion before being available for reutilization in the land of dreams.

## A Split Brain in Dreaming

Visual dreams containing movement are by far the commonest (and 18% of our series were in color). Visual dreams may contain sound, which we sometimes hear as a verbal message that we can easily write down upon waking, even if it does not seem to make sense.

Study of eighty-five recalled auditory dreams gave the following results:

• In 54% of cases a semantic message was easily retained, but it was impossible to recall the face of the messenger. There may have been a telephone involved, or an easily recognized figure (a policeman, a nurse, a priest) *whose face was then utterly forgotten.*

• The messenger could be recognized and recalled in only 20% of cases, usually with the familiar face of a relative, friend, or colleague.

• On the contrary, in 13% of cases the face of the messenger was perfectly well recognized, but *the verbal or written message was totally incomprehensible.* It was in an absolutely foreign language, or a snippet of a phrase that could not be understood, or, in most cases, spoken too quietly to be heard, leading to efforts to have the message repeated.

• Finally, in 13% of cases an unrecognized face was combined with a semantic message that was incomprehensible or foreign.

So, in 67% of cases there was a dissociation between the recognition of the face of a messenger and the recognition of the semantic content of the message. This proportion seems significant. In *La Boutique Obscure* by Georges Perec,[123] which contains 124 transcriptions of recalled dreams without commentary, a similar proportion is found after analysis of the first sixty-four dreams (fifteen cases of dissociation against five).

Here are some examples of dissociation from our series of dream recall and from that of Perec.

1. Precise recall of the semantic content of a message from someone whose face is unknown or forgotten.

• Dream no. 539, June 1972: I am walking in an unfamiliar town, through an inside gallery (like in Milan). I meet M. He is very thin but I recognize him easily. He is with an *unknown woman* who seems to be wearing a black wig. M. walks past me without speaking. The woman leaves him and comes towards me. As she passes she says very loudly, "He loves the thousands of meters of his intestine". I think she is referring to M's love of eating and I am astonished ...

• Dream no. 1305, March 1974: In the USA an *unknown girl*, whose face I cannot recall, gives me the address of a hotel. I can read it in very small writing in her address book. *Lexington. Riverside.* I think it must refer to Riverside Drive in New York, but she tells me in a loud voice, "*Riverside Avenue, 141st Street* ...". It is a hotel costing $5000 a month ...

• Dream no. 2281, May 1977: In an unknown place an unknown girl accompanied by her enormous mother comes up to me. She tells me, "cats do not take their berets off ..."

*From Perec:*

• Dream no. 13, February 1970: I ask what whiskies they have at the bar. They tell me a certain number, using words like "Long John," "Glen ...," "Mac ...," then the word "Chivas" that *they repeat several times*, but deforming it as "Chavaz," "chivelle," etc ...

• Dream no. 16, July 1970: Three men enter the café (*they are obviously cops*). They wander round the room. Perhaps they have not seen me. I breathe a sigh of relief, but one of them comes to sit at my table. "I don't have any papers on me," I say. He is about to get up and go ... but *he says to me very quietly*, "Copulate." I do not understand. He writes the word in the margin of a newspaper *in big black letters*: COPULATE ...

2. Dream recall in which the messenger's face is identifiable but whose message has no semantic value.

• Dream no. 768, December 1972: I meet a friend, B., in Paris. I recognize him but call him Jacques, which is not his name. B. is writing an article that he shows me but *I cannot read what he is writing. Imperceptibly his article becomes a ski race as if I was watching television.*

• Dream no. 1052, July 1973: In a symposium in the USA, M. (whom I recognize perfectly well) presents a communication, but with such a strange accent that I cannot understand him. R. (whom I also recognize easily although I have not seen him for years) waves to me to go closer to M. to be able to understand him better.

• Dream no. 1292, Mach 1974: At a scientific conference I am looking for some slides in my bag before speaking. M. is speaking. I find he looks younger, and he is wearing an electric blue suit. *I cannot hear him. His voice does not reach me because the microphone is not switched on …*

*From Perec:*

• Dream no. 32, November 1970: I am with Z. at the top of some stairs. Elsa Triolet goes by below us … She nods to me. I say to Z., "That's Elsa Triolet." Z. asks me how young I was when she met me and says that she will introduce me to someone who knew me even younger. *But all this is said in such a way that I cannot understand if it will be a man or a woman, or if she means "even younger than me."*

• Dream no. 35, December 1970: Z. comes down, *superbly beautiful.* I lead her into a small, narrow room, like a tube. I tell her that I am leaving her. She says, "But I am going to give you a … (I cannot recall the word: tribe, diploma, secret, seal)."

The existence of this dissociation poses a number of problems. It is now accepted that the recognition of faces (in right-handed people) depends on the right hemisphere and speech or writing on the left. *We might therefore assume that there is a loss of connectivity, at least temporarily, between the two hemispheres during certain dreams.*

This loss of connectivity could have a neurophysiological explanation. Whereas the electrical activity of the great majority of cortical and subcortical neurons increases dramatically during paradoxical sleep, there are two remarkable exceptions.[8] They are the corpus callosum (the enormous bridge of nerve fibers that connects the two hemispheres), and certain parts of the hippocampus (the sea horse–shaped part of the phylogenetically "old" temporal cortex known to be associated with memory). The corpus callosum in fact becomes totally silent, apart from brief bursts during REMs, at least in the cat. At the end of paradoxical sleep, whether followed by normal sleep or by waking up, callosal activity increases immediately. So there seems to be active inhibition of information transfer between the hemispheres during paradoxical sleep. Although there is so far no information on similar callosal activity in primates, or more importantly still, in humans, it is not too bold to assume that the phenomenon of callosal inhibition can occur in dreams. So the difficulty that one has after certain dreams in describing both the semantic message and the face of the messenger could be due to the fact the at the time callosal activity has been temporarily suspended. Experimental proof of this hypothesis is theoretically possible. In the case of recollection of faces, the right hemisphere should be triggered by the right pontine generator. But at the same time pontine nuclei are responsible for excitation of the contralateral (opposite), and inhibition of the ipsilateral (same side), lateral rectus muscle, the tiny muscle that causes the eye to turn outward. Thus the dreamer's eyes should turn to the left when a face is recognized, and to the right when a semantic message is perceived. If dreamers are systematically woken when there is polygraphic evidence of eye deviation in a specific direction, dream recall from different hemispheres should be elicited.

## Paradoxical Sleep and Lucid Dreams

A. I dreamed that I was flying. *I was sure that I was not dreaming. I was sure I was awake* and I was surprised that I had not tried to fly earlier, it was so easy ...

B. I dreamed that I was flying. At that moment *I was sure that I was dreaming* but I was not moving. I watched my own flight in astonishment, without knowing what was to happen. It was an amazing feeling.

These are the two modalities of dream consciousness that one can reveal by waking subjects during dreaming (the flying dream is quite frequent and allows analysis of consciousness because of its strange nature).

Everybody, at least everybody who remembers dreams, remembers a dream like that of A. Its most famous archetype is the dream of Chuang Tzu dreaming that he is a butterfly, or that of the butterfly dreaming that it is Chuang Tzu. The reality of dream consciousness is well summed up in Havelock Ellis's phrase, "Dreams are true while they last. Can we at the best say more of life?"[39] Our dream consciousness reacts like this, as if it were awake. We think that we are not dreaming. It is thus *conscious awareness* because we can ask ourselves if we are dreaming. Dream consciousness is thus similar to that of a hallucinating awake subject. Dream or hallucinatory images triggered by an endogenous system in the brainstem are considered to be real, even if fantastic. Thus the reasoning of conscious awareness during waking is absent. The illusion of reality during dreams has been the subject of numerous commentaries by philosophers. We shall attempt later to sort out some psychophysiological aspects of them.

Type *B* dreams are much rarer (1% or 2% of dream memories). We call them *lucid* dreams. A dream is lucid when the subject, while dreaming, knows he or she is dreaming. This peculiar state allows the dreamer a certain measure of control over the actual unfolding of the dream and a sense of freedom through being able to explore the dream world according to his or her own inclination.

The fact that some people dream knowing all the time that they are dreaming was first noted by Aristotle. Descartes had a series of dreams on a famous night of November 11, 1619, which inspired his vision of a new philosophy and scientific system. The third of his dreams was a lucid dream. Descartes is speaking of himself in the third person[36]: "What is peculiar to remark is that, doubting whether what he had just seen was dream or vision, not only he decided while sleeping that it was a dream, but he made his interpretation before sleep left him ..."

We know that this dream led him to propose a dichotomy between *res immateria* and *res materia* and the phrase, "I think, therefore I am," which was destined to hold up study of the subconscious in France.[154]

More recently lucid dreaming was related at length by the Marquis Hervey de Saint-Denis (1823–1892). In 1867 he published a remarkable work derived from a study of his own dreams: '*Les Rêves et les Moyens de les Diriger*' ("Dreams and How to Direct Them").

Let us consider two recollections of lucid dreams. The first is by Hervey de Saint-Denis, and the second by Frederik van Eeden, a Dutch psychotherapist of the turn of the century.

1. In another dream I see myself on horseback on a fine day, but I am conscious of my real situation, as also the question as to whether I

enjoy full freedom to control my imaginary actions in the dream or not. I say to myself, "This horse is a mere illusion, this countryside that I am crossing a décor, but even if it is not my will that has evoked these images, I feel that at least I have some control over them. I wish to gallop, I gallop; I wish to stop, I stop. Now I see two paths ahead of me. The one on the right seems to plunge into a dense wood; the one on the left leads to a sort of ruined manor. I feel clearly that I have the choice of turning right or left and thus to decide myself if I want to see the birth of associations of ideas and images related to these ruins or with this wood. At first I turn right, then the idea comes to me that it would, in the best interests of my experience, be better to direct such a lucid dream toward the turrets and the keep, because by trying to remember exactly the main details of this architecture I would perhaps be able, upon waking, to recognize the origins of my memories. So I take the path on the left. I dismount at the entrance to a picturesque drawbridge and for the few instants that I still remain asleep I examine very attentively an infinite variety of details great and small: pointed arches, sculpted stones, half-rusted ironwork, fissures and damage in the wall, admiring the minute precision with which all this is engraved before my eyes. However, soon, while I am contemplating the gigantic lock of an old broken door, the objects suddenly lose their color and the distinctness of their contours, like the figures of a diorama when the lamp goes out. I feel I am waking. I open my eyes to the real world, and the glow of my night-light is the only thing that lights me. It is three in the morning.

2. On September 9, 1904, I dreamed that I was standing in front of a table near a window. Various objects were lying on the table. I was fully aware that I was dreaming, and I thought about the experiments I could perform. I began by trying to break a glass by hitting it with a stone. I placed a small glass plate on two stones and hit it with another stone, but in vain. Then I took a fine crystal glass from the table and gripped it in my fist as hard as I could, thinking all the time how dangerous it would be to do that while awake. The glass did not break, but when I looked at it later, it was broken! It had broken as it should have, but a little late, like an actor missing his cue! This gave me the very curious impression of being in a fake world, very well faked, but with small mistakes. So I took the broken glass and threw it out of the window to see if I could hear the noise of the pieces. I heard it very well, and even noticed two dogs running away very naturally. I thought what a good imitation this comedy world was. Seeing a carafe

of Bordeaux on the table, I poured myself some, and noted with perfect clarity, "Well, one can even have conscious sensations of taste in this dream world; this wine tastes perfect!"

We had to await recent work, however, to obtain proof that lucid dreams only occur during paradoxical sleep. In 1985 Stephen LaBerge attempted to analyze his own lucid dreams objectively.[94] He saw the problem as follows. As most of the body is paralyzed during paradoxical sleep, how could a dreamer send a message to say he was dreaming? What could the lucid dreamer do that could be seen and measured by observers? He saw one obvious exception to this muscle paralysis, in that eye movements are in no way hindered during paradoxical sleep. This was, after all, one of the features of 'REM' sleep! So he decided that if he moved his eyes in a recognizable fashion "in the dream," he might be seen to be having a lucid dream by observers. Several subjects were trained to signal by specific combinations of eye and finger movements, or by clenching their fists, all recorded by EMG on the polygraph tracing of their sleep, just when they realized they were dreaming.

Lucid dreams are indeed real dreams. Lucid dreamers have been the subjects of recordings throughout the night with electrodes on the scalp, the orbits, and the muscles. This makes it possible to note the unequivocal appearance of the key signs of paradoxical sleep (which are impossible to simulate). LaBerge was able to make a number of records of periods of lucid dreams during which the coded signal appeared.[53,94,95] His group studied seven subjects, five men and two women, who were known to be capable of lucid dreams, for fifty-two nights. During this study, fifty lucid dreams were recorded in this way. In every case that subjects signaled a lucid dream, it was confirmed as being during a period of paradoxical sleep. The two principal conclusions of this study were that lucid dreaming can occur during paradoxical sleep and that it is possible for lucid dreamers to signal to their environment while continuing to dream. In certain cases dream cognition can be much more reflective and rational than sometimes assumed. This suggested to LaBerge the feasibility of a new approach to dream research: lucid dreamers could participate in experiments allowing precise psychophysiological correlations by marking the exact time of dream events.

I must confess that for a long time I did not believe in lucid dreams. However, four times in the last three years I have enjoyed the extraordinary subjective experience of watching the unfolding of dream images that I could not influence but which I knew full well were part of a dream. An *ego*, conscious of being conscious, and awake, is dreamed up by an unconscious self who cannot interfere, except by stopping the event by the slightest movement. The neurobiological interpretation of such phenomena is totally obscure.

Thus, semiological, linguistic, and neuropsychological study of longitudinal series of recalled dreams in a large sample of people from all backgrounds, normal and pathological, could furnish information complementary to that derived from elaborate stories of dreams told after a long delay on the psychoanalyst's couch.

While we await the establishment of "dream banks," I should like to offer to psychoanalysts, who are experts at playing on words, the following message from the goldfish bowl of sleep that we call dreams, delivered to me by a faceless messenger just before waking recently: *The genome only plays ball with the unconscious.*

# 4

# Oneiric Behavior

The sleep-wake cycle is part of the circadian rhythm of activity and rest, the value of which we all appreciate. The similarity of certain sleep mechanisms to those of hibernation places this form of rest in the general context of an organism's energy-saving mechanisms.

Although we may subjectively feel the benefits of a good night's sleep in the quality of our waking life (our level of attentiveness and our memory), we do not yet know the biological basis of brain fatigue, nor how it appears during prolonged waking, nor how it disappears. From recordings of their electrical activity, we know that neurons do not rest in the strict sense, but have different forms of activity during sleeping and waking. What is more, as we have seen, sleeping is not a uniform activity: several sleep states exist, notably a sleep state that corresponds to that mysterious activity, the dream. Why do episodes of dreaming appear periodically during sleep, episodes of a state of brain activity as different from sleeping as sleeping is from waking? Dreaming may not appear to be a biological necessity; indeed it seems to disturb the body's recuperation from fatigue. What is more, the phenomenon of

Originally published in *Pour la Science* (1989) 59:136–152.

dreaming disturbs the neurobiologist who could do without this added complication in his bid to decipher brain function!

As we have seen, the executive structures of paradoxical sleep have a particular organizational feature: the command systems for postural atonia are near neighbors of the PGO generators in the pons (see chapter 2). If we wish to observe the gestures of oneiric behavior we must make lesions in the atonia command systems to release the block on the body muscles. The proximity of these systems to the PGO generators makes the operation very delicate. In our laboratory Jean-Paul Sastre took several years to complete successful operations in a dozen cats and analyze in detail the repertoire of their oneiric behavior.[139] Either the lesion of the atonia command neurons was too small, leading to recovery of the atonia and the disappearance of oneiric behavior, or the lesion was too extensive and encroached on the PGO generator, thus spoiling the behavioral pattern. The success rate is still relatively low and we shall have to perfect specific biochemical lesioning of the atonia system using neurotoxins, for the technique of making surgical lesions is too risky.

**Oneiric Behavior in Cats**

We can be sure that human subjects dream during paradoxical sleep, for they can describe their recalled dreams, but how can we wake a cat during paradoxical sleep and ask it questions? We cannot, but the discovery and analysis of oneiric behavior would lead us to believe that cats do dream. Oneiric behavior was first described in Lyon in 1965[76,79] and has since been mainly studied in our laboratory and that of Adrian Morrison in Philadelphia.[63] Jean-Paul Sastre's work in our laboratory has no rival in the precision of its ethological descriptions.[141]

We have compared the PGO generator to a pacemaker. To employ a more fanciful image, it is like a conductor directing the neurons in the cerebral orchestra. The music made by this orchestra would then be oneiric activity. Oneiric behavior would be an orchestral concert on television without the sound.

In chapter 2 we examined the neuronal nuclei responsible for muscle atonia during paradoxical sleep, and the inhibitory system descending from them to block excitation of motor neurons in the spinal cord. We predicted what might happen if we were to produce a bilateral lesion as precisely as possible (not an easy thing) in these nuclei or in the descending pathway. There would be nothing to stop excitation of the spinal cord during dreaming. We could then observe oneiric behavior, the expression of activity in cortical and subcortical motor systems triggered by the brainstem PGO generator.

Our experimental method has enabled us to relate different patterns of behavior to electrical activity in the brain. An animal is placed in a large Plexiglas cage that allows it great freedom of movement. Its behavior is recorded continuously by means of a video camera. At the same time the electrical activity of the brain and the muscles are displayed on a polygraph. The behavioral patterns and the brain activity are then mixed and displayed on a single screen. The same sequence can be reprojected in slow motion to study possible correlation between peculiarities of PGO activity and movements of the eyes, head, or limbs.

The extraordinary phenomenon of oneiric behavior can be summarized as follows.

After the brainstem lesions, there is no obvious motor or behavioral disturbance during waking. Slow wave sleep is normal. In contrast, paradoxical sleep diminishes over eight to ten

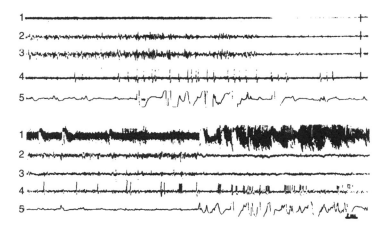

**Figure 14**
(Top) On these recordings we can see the beginning of a period of paradoxical sleep with disappearance of muscle activity (1), acceleration of cortical activity (2, 3), the appearance of PGO activity (4), and rapid eye movements (5). (Bottom) After a lesion in the locus ceruleus alpha, leaving most of the PGO systems intact, the animal demonstrates phases of oneiric behavior with its characteristic signs for several months. Muscle activity increases (1) during dreaming (2–5). We presume that body movements reflect the contents of the dream.

days, after which the whole range of oneiric behavior appears. Following a phase of slow wave sleep during which postural tone may be almost abolished, cortical activation typical of paradoxical sleep begins. The cerebral cortex has fast electrical activity similar to that in waking, while the visual cortex receives endogenous PGO signals from the brainstem that could be a basis for visual imagery (figure 14). Just as the first PGO waves appear, the sleeping cat opens its eyes and raises its head, "looking" upward and sideways instead of lying on the floor in a state of atonia. This pattern of orientation of the head in space and "visual exploration" is a *consistent* feature, but is *paradoxical*: the cat turns its head to the right but looks to the left and vice versa. It seems to pursue some imaginary object moving through space in front of it with its head and eyes. However, the animal does not really see, as can be demonstrated by trying various visual stimulations that elicit absolutely no following reaction. Next come various, but *unpredictable*, stereotyped behavioral patterns that we can attempt to classify into various sequences.

The animal may get up suddenly and begin to walk around its cage as if wanting to explore it. At other times its posture resembles that used in hunting: it behaves as if it could see a mouse, advancing slowly, its head held forward and downward as it pursues its imaginary prey. Sometimes the cat adopts a typical stalking posture, almost immobile with one forepaw slightly raised. It may run after its oneiric prey, stopping to play with it in the characteristic way of a cat that has caught a mouse.

More rarely there are licking or grooming movements. Sometimes a cat licks its coat or its paws, but more often the floor of its cage as if it might be thirsty. This licking is never goal-directed. If you place a piece of adhesive tape on a cat's coat while it is awake it will lick it continuously to remove it, but dream licking is not even directed toward the offending object. Likewise, we have never observed grooming of the face and whiskers with the help of the front paws during oneiric behavior.

We also see two sorts of attack behavior. In the first, *predatory aggression*, the behavior is typified by single or repeated paw strokes toward an imaginary target in front. These may culminate in a movement when the cat uses both front paws to try to capture some imaginary object, sometimes accompanied by gnashing of the teeth. The paw movements may be less violent, as if just touching something or playing. The second pattern is of *aggressive attack*, in the form of paw movements, often directed into the void, with the ears flattened backward and the mouth open ready to bite. The cat seems to be fighting an imaginary enemy.

Another behavioral pattern is that of fear, typified by a general movement of retreat of the whole body as if ready to flee. This pattern ends in a characteristic defensive posture with the back legs flattened against the floor, the ears pulled backward, and the tail slightly raised. This attitude can evolve toward another, just as spectacular, behavior, that of rage, a state full of apparently emotional components. The back is arched, the ears pulled back, the hairs of the back and even of the tail stand up, and the mouth is open as if to bite.

Of note is the fact that these attitudes of aggressive attack, fear, or rage are never accompanied by sounds, as is the case during waking. The only sounds accompanying the cat's oneiric behavior are a few weak and plaintive mews during the phase of visual exploration. We have never noticed the characteristic sound of pleasure, purring.

We have never observed any attitude with sexual components, either in males (erection) or in females (lordosis). Equally, we have never seen shivering, panting, vomiting, or sneezing during oneiric behavior.

Even if it is hungry, the cat will not go to a piece of meat offered to it. It is temporarily blind, and also deaf because it does not react to auditory stimuli. It is entirely under the control of an endogenous system that has taken over its brain and forced it into a dream world.

The sequence of these different patterns of behavior follows no fixed order, apart from the obligatory visual exploration at the beginning. Each animal, however, seems to have a relatively constant proportion, averaged over a week, of different elements in its repertoire, but we have never managed to relate an individual's repertoire to its waking behavior. Curiously enough, those cats that had a large aggressive component in their oneiric behavior were never aggressive toward their experimenters when awake.

It is easy to see that oneiric behavior is an intrinsic phenomenon, but numerous problems remain to be resolved. The absence of reaction to visual and auditory stimuli is understandable: it reflects the complete or partial block of visual and auditory inputs demonstrated during paradoxical sleep. So it is obvious that these behavioral patterns are *aimless*.

Oneiric attack is different from attacking a prey during waking, or from behavior elicited by stimulating the hypothalamus, when an animal may attack any object (the experimenter's hand, for example) but never attacks thin air. The only behavior to which it bears some resemblance is play, such as when a kitten runs after a leaf or attacks an imaginary enemy. As Piaget noted, dreams resemble a "game" inside the brain.

A relationship between different oneiric behavioral patterns and PGO activity is probable, but very difficult to analyze. On the one hand the almost random volleys of PGO activity are hardly compatible with any attempt at semantics. On the other, the complexity of "fight or flight" behavior, involving an almost unlimited number of muscles, does not allow us to analyze in detail how activity of the different muscles may be related to PGO activity. Only the aimless "visual" orientation pattern at the beginning of oneiric behavior is relatively easy to correlate with the PGO "code."

Even if we accept a relationship, at least an indirect one, between activity of the PGO generator and various patterns of oneiric behavior, it still remains to be determined at what level of the brain they originate, where they are elaborated further, and where they go. We are as ignorant on that subject as neurophysiologists studying stereotyped behavioral patterns during waking in response to external or internal stimulation. They know of the probable importance of the amygdala (a nucleus in the temporal lobe closely related to affective behavior; see figure 1), the hypothalamus, and even a locomotor area near the PGO generator, so might these be involved in oneiric activity?

### Oneiric Behavior and Waking Behavior

For the most part, everyday waking behavior is related to one object and one aim, as in the classic stimulus-response concept of behaviorists. In some cases, the trigger stimulus can be minimal if internal motivation is high. It is possible to set off attack behavior by stimulating the brain areas we just mentioned (the amygdala, the hypothalamus, or the brainstem). These attacks are once again directed at a specific object, even an illogical one such as the hand of the experimenter, a dead animal, or a decoy. During playful behavior in young animals the object attacked is also often not a real prey: it may be a dead leaf or a ball of wool, but most of the time one may consider that all attack behavior, or flight or grooming, is directed toward an object in the outside environment.

On the other hand, oneiric behavior is never directed toward an external object: the animal cannot perceive any external stimuli even if they are present. There is filtering of information during paradoxical sleep, either peripherally (by using the tiny muscles of the middle ear to deaden sounds, for instance) or at central relays. This filtering is in part responsible for the raised threshold for waking up, and probably contributes to leaving a free hand to an endogenous program triggered by the pontine generator. It is thus not possible to follow the usual route from the stimulus to the response of the organism to explain the varied activation of motor structures during oneiric behavior. So we must seek the cause of these behavioral patterns in the brain, and in particular in the conductor of the orchestra, PGO activity.

The first hypothesis to explain oneiric behavior was a theory of "scanning" the dream image—which led to the concept of "pseudohallucinatory" behavior, a term we used for oneiric behavior in the early days. As PGO activity invaded the visual system we supposed that it was responsible for hallucinations containing the dream images. If that had been the case the cat would indeed have manifested exploratory and attack behavior if the PGO activity had conjured up the image of a bird or a mouse. But we had to abandon this hypothesis very quickly. Study of latency between the arrival of signals in the visual cortex and eye movements revealed a paradox. In the alert, awake animal the retinal signals provoked by a target object arrive in the visual centers before pursuit eye movements begin (the cause precedes the effect). In contrast, in the dreaming animal the beginning of eye movements *coincides with* or *precedes* the arrival of the endogenous nonretinal signal (the PGO activity) in the visual cortex. It is obviously impossible that the effect (exploratory eye movements) should precede the cause (visual hallucinations). What is more, if eye movements in dreams are related to oneiric images, how can we explain that they already exist during active sleep in the fetal guinea pig, or in the newborn kitten while it is still blind? We must therefore concede that a cerebral system programs or selects the dream imagery and the eye-orientation response *at the same time*. Synaptic delay can explain the latency between a brainstem generator and the arrival of information in the oculomotor nuclei and the visual cortex.

Taken together these data suggest the following hypotheses:

• Oneiric behavior is merely the triggering of organized, complex, automatic behavior without dream images (the cat would then act like an automaton or Descartes' machine-animal), or
• there is sensory excitation (especially visual) at the same time as adaptive phenomena relevant to dream images (attack, flight, pursuit).

This latter hypothesis would force us to accept a fundamental difference between sensorimotor organization in dream consciousness and that of visual perception during waking.

The hallucination hypothesis had, then, to be abandoned, but the role of PGO activity still remains a pivotal feature because its suppression (e.g., by a lesion in the generator) abolishes oneiric behavior. So another theory is now being tested, implicating an endogenous program based on PGO activity (figure 15). This theory can be summarized as follows. The spontaneously active PGO generator neurons can be modulated by the cerebral cortex. They are normally inhibited by the arousal system, as we have already seen in chapter 2 (the noradrenergic brake from the locus ceruleus), and at the beginning of sleep by the raphe system (the serotoninergic brake). When both these brakes are released in a cat with a lesion in the atonia command nuclei, PGO activity triggers directly movement of the head and eyes as the first phase of visual exploration of the dream world. Then, the arrival of PGO information in other structures (such as the amygdala) triggers other stereotyped behavior like attack, rage, or grooming. Indeed, Barry Jacobs and Denis McGinty[72] have demonstrated that amygdala cells in the cat, which respond selectively to mewing during waking, are also active during some periods of paradoxical sleep. It is

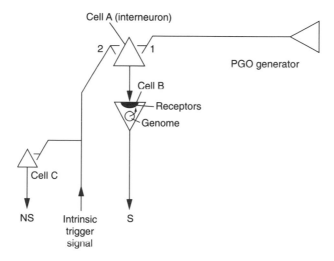

**Figure 15**
Theoretical model of endogenous programming during paradoxical sleep. An interneuron (A) recognizes an intrinsic trigger signal (2) at its first presentation. This interneuron also receives information from the PGO generator during paradoxical sleep (1). It also excites receptors on neuron B during sleep. These receptors depend on protein synthesis controlled by the genome of neuron B. They must receive periodic stimulation from the interneuron in order to remain active. If such "validation" has taken place, the intrinsic signal can trigger the chain of specific reactions (S). If not, the signal will only set off nonspecific reactions (NS), such as attention and arousal, from neuron C which is kept in a constant state of excitement by various environmental stimulations during waking.

out of the question that motor programming of these complex behavioral patterns could be only in the pons, because an animal in which all the brain in front of the pons has been removed is only capable of elementary patterns of behavior during paradoxical sleep, such as walking or running movements. At the same time that these "subprograms" are released, PGO activity can also probably excite certain sensory systems.

So there is *simultaneous* motor programming and excitation of certain sensory integration areas; the motor sequence is not *secondary* to sensory stimulation as was suggested by the hallucination hypothesis.

The central problem with this theory is the nature of the "program." Does it depend on events during the waking period preceding sleep, or does it rather depend on genetic memory? It is still difficult to answer this question but indirect arguments tend to support the second hypothesis. Remember that during ontogenesis, and even in utero, the motor program is expressed by eye movements, and in newborn animals by suckling behavior and "smiles."

As we have seen earlier, mice are the ideal dreaming animals on which genetic experiments can be performed. Jean-Louis Valatx, Raymond Cespuglio, and their colleagues[21] have shown that certain strains of inbred mice manifest patterns of eye movements that are different from those of other strains reared in the same environment (figure 9). Hybrids of the two strains show intermediate patterns. In view of the direct relationship between activity in the PGO generator and rapid eye movements, it seems that the code of PGO activity can be genetically determined. Of course, it is important to know if oneiric behavior in different strains of mice, or of hybrids, is different, but such experiments have not yet proved possible.

Finally, the role of events preceding sleep does not appear to be determinant. It does not seem possible to influence to any extent the pattern of oneiric behavior in a cat by modifying its waking activities: for instance, fasting for two days does not alter the proportion of attack sequences.

Thus, the hypothesis that a cat dreams of actions characteristic of its own species (lying in wait, attack, rage, flight, fright, pursuit) during its paradoxical sleep is quite plausible, although difficult to refute anyway. Certain mechanisms studied in cats during paradoxical sleep can be extrapolated, with reservation, to humans, especially since human oneiric behavior has been described.

## Oneiric Behavior in Humans

In 1986 Carlos Schenck and his colleagues at the University of Minnesota described a syndrome during human sleep resembling oneiric behavior in the cat.[142] It was characterized by:

• a variable reduction in muscular atonia (in particular the chin muscles, as identified by EMG);
• an extraordinary increase in limb activity (spasms, contractions);
• increased number and force of rapid eye movements.

Polygraph recordings confirmed that these phenomena only occurred during paradoxical sleep.

The syndrome was identified in men 67 to 72 years old, and in one woman aged 60, in studies lasting between four months and six years. The woman suffered from a broken-up sleep pattern and manifested oneiric behavior without violent features. In contrast, the men slept continuously, but each manifested aggressive behavior during dreaming, culminating in injuries to their wives and themselves.

In one sequence of such behavior recorded on video cassette one can observe stereotyped movements of the hands, with searching and grasping gestures, blows delivered with the fists and the feet, and vocalization, all seemingly closely related to the contents of their dreams.

The association of dreaming with sleep behaviors was reported directly by (3) patients and was inferred by the spouses of (2 other) patients. Dream processes consisted of mental alertness or hyperalertness; vivid perception, particularly in the visual sphere; frequent motor hyperactivity of the dream characters, including the dreamer; variable emotional experiences; and complex and sometimes bizarre sequences of events, which among the four men often entailed aggressive acts.[142]

The following is one example of an observation of a patient during a polygraph recording in the laboratory.

A behavioral sequence commences with a REM and consists predominantly of right arm shaking and pounding followed by a pause, which is terminated by further right arm pounding, then flexion of that arm as the patient turns toward his left side while making an abortive effort to lift himself up from the bed. When an examiner appears 20 s later, the patient reports having just dreamed of holding a dog or cat in his right arm to restrain it from jumping away, but when it escaped he turned to his left side in an unsuccessful attempt to capture it.[142]

In another dream, a patient was struggling with a dangerous animal and woke when he injured himself while trying to run away. In yet another he was trying to strangle his wife; the emergency treatment used by this patient was to sleep in a different room! A more sophisticated therapy was proposed by the authors, apparently with success: the administration of benzodiazepines. When this regimen was stopped, the symptoms recurred immediately.

We should note that the slow wave sleep of these subjects was devoid of any aggressive behavior, although three of them manifested chronic myoclonic episodes, the muscle spasms that are typical of some forms of epilepsy.

In the subjects studied there was no present or previous history of psychiatric problems, but in four of them a close correlation was discovered between the onset of their oneiric behavior and the development of neurological disease: olivo-ponto-cerebellar degeneration, polyneuritis (Guillain-Barré syndrome), meningeal hemorrhage, and a nonspecific degenerative condition.

**Table 1**
Very schematic table of the principal neurobiological variables observed during waking, sleeping, and dreaming in the cat

|  | Waking | Slow Wave Sleep | Paradoxical Sleep |
|---|---|---|---|
| Cortical electrical activity | Fast | Slow | Fast ($=$) |
| Glucose consumption in visual cortex | Increased | Decreased | Increased ($=$) |
| Oxygen consumption in visual cortex | No increase | Decreased | ? Should increase (not yet confirmed) |
| Brain temperature | Increased | Decreased | Decreased, then increased |
| Eye movements | Follow a target Take place after a retinal signal reaches the cortex | Absent | Triggered by PGO system ($\#$) Precede or are simultaneous with PGO signal reaching the cortex ($\#$) |
| Postural tone | Increased | Decreased | Absent ($\#$) |
| Activity of monoaminergic cortical activating systems | Increased | Decreased | Absent ($\#$) |
| Activity of pyramidal system | Increased | Decreased | Increased ($=$) |
| Activity of PGO generator | Absent | Absent | Highly increased ($\#$) |

Note: $=$ implies a similarity between waking and dreaming; $\#$ implies a difference. (See Orem and Barnes.[121])

So we can establish the following synchronous correlations between an objective neurobiological state (paradoxical sleep) and "mental" phenomena.

- In humans: paradoxical sleep ↔ dream ↔ oneiric behavior
- In the cat: paradoxical sleep ↔ oneiric behavior ↔ dream

These correlations enable us to summarize in table 1 the similarities (=) and the differences (#) between certain neurophysiological events observed during waking, sleeping, and "dreaming" in the cat.

Certain overall conditions are common to attention and dreaming (and absent during sleep). However, it is obvious that brain function is different during waking and dream consciousness, for many brainstem systems are active during waking, whereas they remain inactive or inhibited during dreaming (and vice versa).

# 5

## Sleep, the Other Side of the Spirit

Sleep and spirit. Sleep and mind. The two phenomena seem contradictory. On the one hand the resemblance of sleep and death, exemplified by Hypnos and Thanatos, the twin brothers of Greek mythology, and on the other hand the spirit, the mind, which for me means higher nervous activity, as during waking. It means consciousness.

It is probable that this contradiction existed at the origin of the concept of spirit. Imagine the first hominids sheltering in a cave in East Africa. They already use a rudimentary language and they think, but they do not yet *know* that they think. One of them wakes after a dream and recounts how, during the night, he left the cave and flew like a bird. His companions look at him, stupified and incredulous. Then the same phenomenon is repeated, over and over.

The human mind had to choose between two concepts of dreams: the errant soul leaving the body to abandon itself to a nightly wandering, or the activity of gods and demons visiting the sleeper with their revelations (see chapter 2).[18]

Of course, it is not up to the neurobiologist to retrace the history of dreaming, this first insight into the subconscious dis-

Originally published by the Pontifical Council for Health Services in *Dolentium hominum* (1991) 16: 60–68.

covered long before the concepts of conscious and subconscious in cognitive and affective life. The neurobiologist's still impossible task is to try to explain, in the light of our present knowledge, the role of the mind in the machinations of the night.

First we must determine our position with respect to the different "schools" that have studied consciousness, for on this depends our definition of the mind.

Neither behaviorism, which avoids the problem of mind and consciousness, nor functionalism, which is only interested in performance and which might well accept that a computer is conscious, nor panpsychism, is appropriate for our study. In the absence of proof of a concept of external nonmaterial influences acting on the brain in contradiction to the laws of thermodynamics, I, for the moment, subscribe to the school that we might call "psychoneural identity," clearly opposed to Cartesian dualism in its original form or in its more recent developments.

As I said, for me, the spirit is the conscious mind, the result of higher nervous activity: the perception, or apperception, of the environment, the representation of absent figures (mental imagery) permitting complex responses and communications with our peers. In short, in humans, there are primary consciousness ("I think"), conscious awareness or superior order consciousness, ("I think that I think"), and the unconscious ("I acted without thinking"). I accept that certain aspects of consciousness can exist in all warm-blooded animals, including birds (the Gabon gray parrot can recall 1200 words, more than a child of 5 years of age.[60] Self-consciousness (recognizing one's face in a mirror) emerges in the chimpanzee, but not in the gorilla. Conscious awareness is probably restricted to waking man ("I am conscious of being conscious") and to dreamers. In the latter case, as we shall soon see, it can be subject to strange distortions.

The different synchronic operational modes of consciousness are broadened by a diachronic component related to memory. In general we remember our thoughts and our conscious acts easily, and associations of ideas enable us to discover the origin of some unconscious acts.

## The Waking Mind

Before tackling the problem of consciousness during sleep we must consider what we observe when a man, or a cat, performs conscious acts during waking (being attentive, for example). We can only consider them as phenomena, for no one has yet been able to identify any adequate or necessary *causality* involved in consciousness.

Three major phenomena seem to accompany consciousness:

1. It requires the integrity of certain cerebral cortical areas, especially in the parietal lobe. There is no evidence of perception in patients with widespread cortical lesions.

2. Cortical integrity is, however, not enough. There must be a certain level of excitation of the numerous modules that constitute the basic cortical functional units. This excitation, the arousal reaction, is seen as specific cortical electrical activity recorded from the human scalp or from electrodes placed directly in the cortex in animals. Arousal, whether produced by signals from the external environment or signals generated by the cortex itself (mental images), is not a purely cortical phenomenon but needs activity in subcortical systems. These systems, from the medulla to the hypothalamus, release neurotransmitters (catecholamines, serotonin, acetylcholine, peptides, and histamine) that activate the cortical areas according to complex hierarchies and patterns.

3. Consciousness is accompanied by specific energy transformations that can be demonstrated with a positron camera (see chapter 1), for the cortical modules consume more glucose,

and have increased blood flow, when active. However, there seems to be an uncoupling between glucose and oxygen consumption such that the cortex can use the anaerobic energy pathway, producing lactate, during attention.[49]

In summary, waking consciousness needs a degree of cortical integrity associated with excitatory activity in the brainstem. This process implies an increase in energy in the form of glucose metabolism, which can be anaerobic.

## Sleep States and the Mind

We have already seen in the great majority of warm-blooded animals (birds and mammals) the two states of sleep characterized by behavioral, electrophysiological, and metabolic differences: slow wave sleep and paradoxical sleep. We must therefore study the relationship of these two states with the mind.

Slow wave sleep is characterized by the disappearance of two major features that accompany waking consciousness.

1. First, cortical electrical activity slows and is encroached upon by spontaneous activity, referred to as "spikes," of thalamic origin. We suppose that at this time inhibition at the thalamocortical level prevents conscious perception. As the depth of sleep increases, high-voltage slow waves appear, originating in some unknown cortical mechanism.

2. Sleep is also accompanied by a marked reduction in glucose and oxygen consumption by the cortex,[50] while energy reserves are stored in glial cells in the form of glycogen.[57,89]

## The Mind during Slow Wave Sleep

A first remark is called for, originally expressed by the Cambridge Platonist Ralph Cudworth in 1678 in reply to René Descartes.[28]

Cudworth believed in an unconscious vital energy of which an individual was not aware. He pointed out that philosophers who attributed the essence of the soul to reflection, and the essence of reflection to consciousness, could not maintain that the human soul in deep sleep was never devoid of explicit consciousness. If such were so, their own philosophical principles would imply that they would cease to exist. He was certain that our soul was not always conscious of what it contained. The sleeping geometrist did not lose his geometrical theorems, just as the sleeping musician continued to preserve all his musical aptitudes and melodies.

Thus we have known for a long time that memory can survive deep sleep (and it can even persist in the face of a total absence of cerebral electrical activity during hypothermia). What happens to consciousness, perception, or apperception of the environment? It has been shown that learning ceases completely during sleep and that "sleep learning" is an illusion, even if sleep *after* learning can be beneficial. Data concerning consciousness during sleep come essentially from human studies, by waking sleeping subjects under EEG control. Such experiments have been carried out over the last forty years in numerous laboratories. The results show clearly that if subjects are woken suddenly during the sleep period preceding the first dream, most are incapable of recalling the slightest memory, and often cannot even guess how long they were asleep, which seems to indicate a suspension of consciousness, even the consciousness of being asleep. The snorer does not know he has been snoring. In 30% of cases, however, it is possible to obtain recall of some abstract thought, completely different from dream images. The subject thinks he or she has dreamed, but is incapable of describing the dream.[29]

## The Problem of Sleepwalking

Sleepwalking is considered as rare but not pathological and 10% of cases occur in infants and adolescents of less than 15 years. It occurs during slow wave sleep, as proved by telemetric EEG recordings.[54] A sleepwalker can get up, open a door, and fetch food. When woken suddenly, the sleepwalker does not know why he or she is up and has no memories of the episode.

Sleepwalking is thus a good example of the absence of psychoneural correlation that should teach the neurobiologist a lesson in humility: in spite of the presence of slow cortical waves (and therefore presumably in the absence of cortical activity that we consider a condition of consciousness), we observe complex goal-directed behavior. For a behaviorist this could suggest something similar to waking consciousness, but close analysis reveals no memory of sleepwalking behavior.

After this first analysis, neurobiologists and clinical neurophysiologists must admit that the relationships between sleep and consciousness are ambiguous and that the following preliminary conclusions are plausible.

During slow wave sleep preceding the first phase of dreaming, there is no evidence for the existence of conscious awareness—consciousness of sleeping. No one can say, "I think I am asleep," and even less, "I think that I think I am asleep."

It is possible that a short period of waking during sleep (accompanied by cortical activation) is enough to allow access to primary consciousness ("I think that I thought of something").

The sleepwalker's perception, enabling the opening and closing of a door, is a good example of unconscious perception. Sleepwalkers, even adults, never say, "I think that I am sleepwalking," and they never remember their exploit when they are woken. We must therefore accept that unconscious perception, not accompanied by integration into memory, can sometimes exist in the absence of cortical activation during sleep.

## Dream Consciousness

The question whether we only dream during paradoxical sleep still provokes much discussion. In the last few years, many people have asked me about the current state of sleep and dream research. I always emphasize the long controversy between the partisans of continuous dreaming during sleep and those who defend the hypothesis of dreaming being the subjective equivalent of paradoxical sleep. This controversy relates directly to a basic problem that still remains unresolved: what is the relationship between the electrical activity of the brain and waking or sleeping consciousness? There is much relevant work on this subject, and I should like to refer to some of it. The more inquisitive of you will be able to go directly to the source to decide which trend to follow!

There are divergent theories. According to one that was in the minority in the 1970s, mental activity continues throughout the whole of sleep. This concept is a heritage of Freud's idea that *throughout our whole sleeping state we know just as certainly that we are dreaming as we know that we are sleeping.*[13,52,104]

The second theory recognizes the large number of dreams during paradoxical sleep and their rarity during slow wave sleep. The two theories are slowly diverging with the result that dream research is now conducted by groups that have little mutual contact.

Let us try to summarize as objectively as possible the evolution of these ideas in the last decade, beginning with the theory

that there is continuous mental activity during sleep according
to which

> Neuronal activity patterns in many brain areas are qualitatively dif-
> ferent in REM and NREM ("non-REM") sleep. However, there are no
> qualitative differences between NREM and REM mentation report.
> The startling conclusion of this syllogism is that the striking NREM/
> REM difference in neuronal firing must not involve the neural systems
> that can affect the quality of conscious experience. A partial explana-
> tion of this paradox may lie in the fact that the most extreme NREM/
> REM differences in neuronal activity are found in hard wired systems,
> including brainstem centers and primary sensory and motor cortex.
> Thus there may be a dissociation of the brain centers that mediate
> consciousness from those involved in perception and movement.[43]

This theory refutes a direct equivalence between dreaming
and paradoxical sleep, but also leads to the conclusion that
*there is no correlation between mental activity and the EEG.*

Of course, there is still a hypothesis, which has never been
seriously studied, that memories of mental activity on waking
up during any stage of sleep could represent memories created
during the waking process itself.

I frankly support the theory that we do not dream all night,
as do William Dement and Alan Hobson and most neurophysiologists. I am rather surprised that publications about
dream recall during slow wave sleep increase in number each
year. Further, the classic distinction established in the 1960s
between "poor" dream recall, devoid of color and detail, during slow wave sleep, and "rich" recall, full of color and detail,
during paradoxical sleep, is beginning to disappear.[13] I believe
that dream recall during slow wave sleep could be recall
from previous paradoxical sleep. It is also probable that
dreamlike activity may occur while falling asleep (stage 1) in
some people. As waking consciousness fades away it may
induce a dreamlike state akin to certain hypnotic hallucina-

tions. Indeed, similar hallucinations can occur during some forms of anesthesia.

It would be interesting to catalog dream recall, if there is any, during the first deep sleep cycle (stages 2, 3, and 4) *before* the first period of paradoxical sleep and compare it with recall during subsequent cycles *after* a period or periods of paradoxical sleep.

The concept of a precise relationship between the EEG and mental activity is so important that we ought perhaps to use pharmacological methods to verify it. I once used to treat cataplectic narcoleptics with imipramine. I remember one patient who recorded his dreams every day, building up a library of thousands of dreams. He had noticed that increasing the dose of imipramine led to a total absence of dreams for several weeks. If we then reduced his dose radically there was a "rebound" in the number of dreams, up to thirty a night. We know from polygraph records that imipramine suppresses paradoxical sleep. I should very much like to attempt the following experiment. We would make polygraph recordings of sleep in volunteers given a dose of imipramine before going to bed, or just given an inert "placebo." The conditions would have to be strictly controlled and "double blind"—that is, with neither subject nor experimenter knowing what they had taken. We would, of course, have to determine from control recordings what dose suppresses paradoxical sleep just enough. The subjects would be woken every ninety minutes and asked what they were "thinking" about. During placebo nights it is very likely that they would sometimes be woken during paradoxical sleep and sometimes during slow wave sleep. Independent observers examining the polygraph would decide that. In contrast, we can be sure that they would not be woken during paradoxical sleep on imipramine nights. These experiments would be relatively easy to perform and I can see no ethical problem with such an innocuous drug as imipramine.

I accept that *very precise* recall of dreams during imipramine nights, when there would be a total absence of paradoxical sleep all night, would *totally and definitively* refute the hypothesis of an equivalence between paradoxical sleep and dreaming. On the other hand, I admit that the absence of dream recall during imipramine nights would not be an *absolute* proof of such equivalence. Indeed, opponents of that hypothesis could argue that imipramine might suppress dream activity by some unknown mechanism not related to the mechanism by which it stops paradoxical sleep.

I have, for several reasons, never undertaken this experiment. First, I am no longer continuing my hospital practice, and second, the relationship between paradoxical sleep and dreaming is no longer my main preoccupation.

Some great cognitivist thinkers have recently revisited the theory of equivalence between dreaming and paradoxical sleep. The problem of consciousness is very fashionable, and some of these "cogniscientists" penetrated the field of mental activity during sleep when it became "respectable"! Some cognitive physiologists have a profound knowledge of cerebral electrical activity, and have studied its frequencies and topography in vivo and in vitro. Their background has led them to concentrate on brain rhythm, often to the exclusion of other essential features of sleep physiology, such as the effect of neurotransmitters, as well as of ontogenesis and phylogenesis. Rodolfo Llinás and his collaborator[99] proposed a revolutionary idea, almost worthy of a Copernicus. They suggested that it is not paradoxical sleep that needs explaining, but wakefulness. After declaring that "Consciousness and subjectivity are intrinsic properties of the brain" (if not of the brain, then of which other organ?), they affirmed that thalamocortical activity is responsible for consciousness and that "it is the dialogue between the thalamus and the cortex that generates subjectivity." Most people would have subscribed to that concept decades ago if they had been familiar with the language of this dialogue! Then they stated "that wakefulness is nothing other than a dreamlike state modulated by the constraints produced by specific inputs" while REM sleep could be considered as a modified attentive state in which attention is turned away from the sensory input, toward neurons. Thus waking and REM sleep were very similar. So similar "that a possible approach to understanding the nature of wakefulness is to consider it as one element in a category of intrinsic brain functions, in which REM sleep is another element."

If this hypothesis is correct, what about animals that do not have paradoxical sleep? How can they be awake? There is no doubt that we experience consciousness, whether awake or sleeping. So there must be an explanation. Some people see the explanation in the magic number "forty hertz" (forty cycles per second or 40 Hz). To explain consciousness we should realize that activity in widely separate parts of the brain must be synchronized. This synchronization, or temporal binding, between different groups of neurons is achieved by fast electrical activity at 40 Hz. This "gamma" activity can be recorded by magnetoelectroencephalography both during waking and in paradoxical sleep. Where and how gamma activity is generated remains a mystery: the cortex, the thalamus, the amygdala? So dreaming is basically hyperactivity, like being wide-awake. In their long, synthetic article, Llinás and Paré[99] made no reference to the essential differences between activity of, for example, aminergic systems during waking and their total inactivity during dreams.

If the *mechanisms* of waking and dreaming have been explained, what is the *function* of dreaming according to these new explorers of consciousness? It is not related to "noise" coming from the brainstem, as Hobson and McCarley suggested in 1977.[67] Llinás and Ribary[100] proposed a hypothesis based partly on that of Crick and Mitchison[27] (see chapters 1 and 6), that we dream to forget in order not to overload our brain. Indeed, Llinás and Ribary claim that "it often happens that having come to a solution considered adequate, a second may 'pop up' in one's mind at a later time. We may further consider that at the end of the day we may have many such partial computations being performed prior to our falling asleep. The possibility is there that in dreaming we 'download' the other possible solutions and thus prevent the overloading of circuits with the accumulation of an ever-increasing set of ongoing partial solutions as new problems are considered. This particular point of view may be supported in part by the fact that excellent solutions to problems may arise in dreams."

Such a hypothesis could be of use for our cognitivists. But could it be valid for a cat, a rat, or a bird?

It is important to read Llinás and Ribary's article to the end, for they have also found a function for slow wave sleep. "Something quite similar may be said with regard to slow-wave sleep. In this case the very short oscillatory nature of the neuronal rhythmicity observed during this functional state is probably closer to the grooming functions that most animals perform upon finishing a task." As humans do not groom like cats, can we conclude that slow wave sleep fulfills the function of a rocking chair?

Steriade and his colleagues[151] were much more prudent when they discussed the thorny question of the magic frequency of 40 Hz in relation to consciousness and dreaming. "The attraction for this magic frequency ignores the fact that rhythms implicated in attentive processes or produced by optimal sensory signals extend over a rather broad spectrum, from as low as 14 Hz to as high as 80 Hz." So 40 Hz is abandoned. What is more, Steriade's team attacked the concept of *desynchronization* of cortical activity and replaced it with *synchronization*. Then, like most neurophysiologists, they contrasted the synchronization of waking involving aminergic systems with the synchronization of paradoxical sleep in which these systems are inhibited. They were especially careful when considering correlations between cortical EEG activation and consciousness. The correlation between complex variations in fast rhythm and functional states is probable when dealing with very short phenomena, but rather improbable when dealing with global function. Steriade considered that fast rhythms, including 40 Hz, are not necessarily related to higher nervous or mental activity, because they can be found, at least in a transitory fashion, during slow wave sleep.

While Llinás and his colleagues are prisoners of the hypothesis that 40 Hz activity is necessary, and perhaps sufficient, for waking and dreaming consciousness, Steriade, more prudently, left another opening. Fast rhythms vary in frequency and can be found in slow wave sleep. So, could they be responsible for a given mental state during sleep?

Recently Hobson and his colleagues[88] attempted an explanation of the difference between waking and dreaming consciousness according to the degree of modulation by aminergic systems. This approach is related to trying to equate cortical activity with consciousness. This is why I believe that we should again study and compare states of consciousness during slow wave sleep, and even during sleepwalking that we discussed earlier in this chapter.

**Conclusion**

The spirit, or mind, as observed through the window of memory of a sleeper or dreamer who wakes, is obscured by various different concepts of consciousness. We have attempted an explanation in neurobiological terms of the different aspects of consciousness during sleep and dreams, and its similarities and differences compared with waking consciousness. Even if we can see the beginnings of some global psychoneural parallelism, the unknown is still far in advance of our modest knowledge.

However, it seems that one possible path to an understanding of the function of the mind is provided by studying dreams.

# 6

# The Functions of Dreaming

As we have seen, paradoxical sleep, and therefore perhaps dreams, appeared in the course of evolution at the same time as warm-bloodedness. It is difficult to understand how dreaming can provide an evolutionary advantage when it corresponds to a state when the animal is most vulnerable. The dream state is indeed the most dangerous in the triple cycle of sleeping-waking-dreaming because the brain closes the door to the environment, and hence to possible dangers, and opens up to an endogenous program. The fact that only warm-blooded dreamers have survived is a mystery that we must resolve if we wish to make progress in establishing relevant models of the brain. For all these reasons the study of the mechanisms and functions of dreaming was for more than twenty years one of the most active branches of sleep research.

So there are still many unanswered questions, and much work for physicians trying to understand the numerous disturbances of the sleep-wake-dream cycle, and for neurobiologists. However, we cannot yet find a function (or functions) for dreaming on the basis of the mechanisms that we have just discussed—much too briefly. There must exist as many neuro-biological hypotheses about the function of dreaming as there are researchers in the field: the dream as a sentinel, periodically lightening sleep to allow survival in a hostile environment; the dream converting short-term memory to long-term memory; the dream facilitating, or inhibiting, transfer between the right and left hemispheres; the epiphenomenal dream of no significance (like phantasms during waking); the dream for deleting pointless information (*reverse learning*).

The discovery of the physiological basis of dreams represented a new departure in the history of functional theories of dreaming. Before 1960 Freudian theory and psychoanalysis were dominant. After 1960 study of the neurophysiology and natural history of dreaming endeavored to find "why" there were dreams after the innumerable questions or "how" they occurred.

## Before 1960

At the end of the eighteenth century the vocabulary and the concepts of the unconscious entered into German culture. Georg Christoph Lichtenberg[98] was fascinated by his own dreams and conceived the idea that dreams could be "reminiscences of states before the development of individual consciousness." However, people were still more interested in interpreting the "how" of dreams rather than the "why."

A hundred years later, Robert[133] was the first to put forward a theory of the function of dreaming. He imagined dreaming as a *bodily* (somatic) function of elimination of worthless ideas, of which we are only conscious when we react to it. Freud cited him as saying, "Dreams are the excretion of thoughts that have been stifled at birth." A man who was deprived of the possibility of dreaming would go mad after a while, because an enormous mass of incomplete or undeveloped thoughts and superficial impressions would heap up in his brain and stifle the well-developed thought processes preserved in memory. So the dream became the overloaded brain's safety valve. Dreams, therefore, played a role of relief and remedy. Dreaming was not a psychic process but only the awareness of this process of elimination. But this process was not the only one involved in dreaming. Robert added that impressions and thoughts gathered during the day that had not been eliminated could be completed by our imagination and inserted in our memory in the form of "a harmless, imaginative picture."

Freud further interpreted Robert as defining a dream as a somatic process appearing in the mind each night the function of which is to preserve the mind from excess tension and to purge it.[52] A hundred years later Crick and Mitchison[27] introduced a "computer version" of Robert's theory, without citing him in their bibliography (see below).

At the same time Santiago Ramón y Cajal propounded the hypothesis that the brain is composed of individual cells (the neurons), separated from each other, and not of a reticular system as Golgi and others believed. Exner, Freud's physiology professor, published his *Entwurf zu einer physiologischen Erklärung der psychischen Erscheinungen* ("Outline of a Physiological Explanation of Psychic Events") in 1894.[41] He used his own experiments on reflexes to illustrate the concept of *Bahnung* ("facilitation"). At a given intensity a single stimulus does not elicit a reflex response, but if two stimuli follow each other with a short latency, a response will occur. Exner even went so far as to postulate that inhibition could be an active mechanism dependent on specific nervous pathways.

### Freud's Neuronal Model

Also at this time, in 1895, Freud drafted his "Project for a Scientific Psychology."[51] I shall draw material from the well-documented article of McCarley and Hobson[109] concerning the mistaken physiological statements that provided a basis for Freud's psychoanalytical theory and his model for dreams.

Among the elements of Freud's model that conflict with modern concepts are the neurons. "The neurons in Freud's theory do appear structurally rather modern. They are discrete cells with points of contact between them, and Freud was quite correct in assuming some kind of structural specialization at the gaps between cell processes (which we call synapses). Physiology was the problem area, and Freud's principal ideas and the contrasting modern concepts about neurons can be grouped into four categories."[109]

1. Freud's concept was that neurons functioned as *passive* energy stores, in contrast to the modern concept of neurons as *active* cells specialized for transmission of information. His neurons were capable of being filled by greater or lesser amounts of energy that he called *nervous quantity* or *Q'n*. This stored energy was always derived from sources outside neurons. Our modern view is that neurons utilize their own metabolic energy to maintain a difference in electrical potential (*resting* potential) between the outside and inside of the cell. A decrease in this potential causes a discharge that is propagated along the axon to other cells by the release of chemical transmitters at the synapses. Very little energy is needed by neurons for these functions. It was too soon for Freud to know details about electrical potentials in nerves, only discovered in 1910.

2. Freud viewed neurons as conduits of energy from the environment to the brain.

The current neurophysiological conception of sensory receptor neurons is that they act as transducers, that is, they signal the presence of energy (e.g., light, sound, heat, and skin deformation) in the external world. They transduce this energy into a coded form of electrical signal ... The important concept is that the signal indicates the presence of energy but does not conduct the energy itself into the CNS [central nervous system].[109]

3. Freud saw neurons as passive receptors and donors of energy; we now consider neurons as spontaneously active.

Freud held tenaciously to the idea of neurons as sources and sinks of energy ultimately derived from outside the brain; he on no occasion postulated that neurons had their own metabolic energy sources or that they formed self-regulatory networks. This assumption was of critical importance for Freud's neural model, and it led him to place the cause of dreaming outside the brain, since the ultimate sources of energy were also necessarily extracerebral. Dreams originated from somatic or external stimuli. This assumption further committed Freud to a reactive, essentially passive brain and to a model of the psyche that shared these characteristics.[109]

We now know that dreams depend on endogenously generated neural activity.

4. Freud's theory was that neurons were exclusively excitatory, but we now recognize inhibitory neurons. In contrast with Exner, Freud had no place for inhibitory elements in his model. He therefore had recourse to the concept of *diversion* of energy and the formation of *side paths*. Diverted energy could be "discharged" into motor activity.

In contrast, modern concepts of neural function emphasize the importance of inhibition. Freud's idea of "diversion of excitation" led him to conceive of diverted impulses ("repressed wishes") as a continual pressure, often emerging in dreams.

## Structure and Dynamics of Freud's Model

As there were no inhibitory neurons in Freud's model, he was forced to postulate another principle of neuronal energy flux that had no experimental basis at the time, and still does not. He defined three main types of neuron: $\phi$ (phi) neurons, which

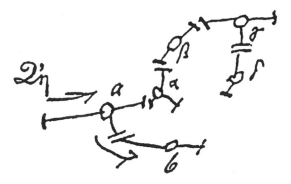

**Figure 16**
Freud's sketch of his concept of the diversion of nervous energy by
"side cathexis." The normal energy flow (indicated by Q'n in Freud's
handwriting) is toward neuron b. Freud postulated that side cathexis
of neuron α would attract Q'n and divert the flow from neuron b.
Freud believed that this side cathexis, or postsynaptic attraction of
energy, for which there is no experimental evidence, was the neuronal
basis for repression.

played a role in perception; $\psi$ (psi) neurons with a psychic
function; and $\omega$ (omega) neurons of consciousness. Figure 16
reproduces Freud's sketch of the direction of energy flow in a
set of neurons. Freud proposed that a charge or *cathexis* in a
neuron would attract Q'n and thus divert nervous energy from
its normal path. Freud spoke of this diversion of energy as
"inhibition," but his concept was distinctly different from the
modern concept of inhibition and based on lack of knowledge
about neuronal function. Freud's concept of *side cathexis*
meant that nervous energy could only be diverted, not really
inhibited, and it made his model nervous system vulnerable to
energy overload. Freud believed that side cathexis was accom-
plished by a specialized set of $\psi$ neurons, which he called the
"ego," a familiar psychological and psychoanalytical concept.

Freud also thought that perceptions of objects that had proved painful in the past were associated with painful affect in the form of excessive energy. These perceptions were linked to "key neurons" which stimulated unpleasurable endogenous sources of Q'n. Figure 16 shows such a neuron (labeled b).

From this neuronal model Freud elaborated a dynamic theory of psychic function. Marc Jeannerod wrote a clear and synthetic treatment of it in his book *Le Cerveau-Machine* ("The Brain Machine"),[74] which will help us understand Freud's concepts.

According to Freud, neurons obey a primary function, which he calls the "principle of inertia." Thanks to a "discharge" mechanism, a neuron disposes of the information that it receives and can maintain itself in a state of nonexcitation ... In certain conditions, however, ... it must learn to store sufficient nervous quantity to satisfy the exigencies of a specific act ...

The primary function is based on the simple notion of a "current" running through the neuron ... Certain neurons, the phi neurons, that function in perception, are easily traversed without retaining anything; others, psi neurons, are resistant and retain nervous quantity. "Memory and probably also psychic processes in general depend on the latter ..."

What is the basis for the difference between the phi and the psi systems? Certainly not morphological criteria, according to Freud, but only the relative "distance" of each neuronal type from the periphery. Phi neurons are in contact with the outside of the body: they are constantly bombarded by large quantities of information and their task is to discharge these quantities as quickly as possible. On the contrary, psi neurons, which Freud localizes in the "gray matter of the brain," remain unconnected with the outside world, only receiving information from phi neurons or from inside the body and, in any case, in much smaller quantity than phi neurons. They can therefore absorb information without too much risk of being overfilled. This energy reserve that is built up in psi neurons allows an intrapsychic circulation of quantities of information of which the degree of accumulation or discharge reflects the state of, respectively, desire or affect. Thus,

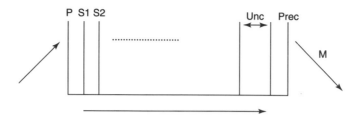

**Figure 17**
Freud's model of the psyche from chapter 7 of *The Interpretation of Dreams*. P, perception system; S1 and S2, memory systems; Unc, unconscious; Prec, preconscious; M, motor system. The arrows indicate the normal direction of energy flow.

according to Freud, free will would consist "of a discharge of the total quantity of psi."

The systems described by Freud obviously derive energy from outside the organism, or at least outside the brain. A small amount of energy is assumed to come from internal sources, represented by the sensation of hunger or sexual desire, for example ... Thus sensations from outside or inside nourish the cerebral machine and give it its excuse for functioning.

## Freud's Model of Dreams

In *The Interpretation of Dreams*, Freud described a psychological model comparable to that of the *Project* (figure 17). His model included three subsystems: mnemic elements, the unconscious (instincts), and the preconscious (psychic elements closely related to consciousness). A "psychic censor" placed between the unconscious and the preconscious acts to block wishes that would be unacceptable to consciousness.

The outline of Freud's dream theory is straightforward. The ego wishes to sleep (why it should is not clear!). It withdraws its "cathexis" from the motor system, resulting in sleep paralysis. The dream process begins when something left over from the waking day's experiences stirs up a "repressed" wish in the unconscious. This force tries to move in the direction of flow in Freud's model (arrows in figure 17) toward the preconscious system. The wish is blocked by the censor, and there is a retreat toward the mnemic elements of the psyche, which are close to the perceptual side. There the "dream" works at symbol formation to disguise the wish with images of those mnemic elements with the closest links to the wish. The disguised wish thus becomes acceptable to the censor and is passed into consciousness. Freud believed that dreams functioned as a *guardian of sleep*, preventing the intrusion of unacceptable wishes into consciousness, with the risk of subsequent arousal. This represents Freud's "wish-fulfillment-disguise" theory of dream generation.

### Freud's Theory of Dreaming in the Light of the Neurophysiology of Paradoxical Sleep

Theories about dreams have shorter and shorter lives and it would be unjust, a hundred years later, to scrutinize Freudian theory in the light of the neurophysiology of paradoxical sleep as we conceive it now. However, I shall once again cite the critique of McCarley and Hobson, with which I entirely agree. I would not have added this critique had there not still been articles defending the Freudian theory of dreaming appearing under the name of certain psychoanalysts, claiming that it is "confirmed by modern neurophysiology." This is a claim I wish to dispel, and McCarley and Hobson[109] give me conclusive support in this!

Freud believed that the dreaming state (D) and dreaming were initiated and powered by the combination of the day residue (certain memories from the day) with the energy contained in a repressed unconscious wish (*see table 4, item 3*). It can now be categorically stated that there is *no* experimental support whatsoever for Freud's theory of D-state generation. Instead, modern investigations point to autochthonous, periodic, and motivationally neutral activation of pontine generator neurons as the cause of the D-state.

The rhythmic state-generation property of these pontine brain stem cells points to other fundamental difficulties with Freud's CNS model, since he nowhere postulated autochthonously active and autochthonously regulated neural systems or their counterpart. The simple conclusion is that Freud's theory regarding the lack of autochthonous activity and the lack of regulation and endogenous energy for the brain must be abandoned. This is not to suggest that day residue material or motivationally important themes do not enter into dream content; they may do so, but neither is a causal factor in the dream process.

There is no need to postulate the repression of Qn (or of wishes, if one prefers this label for neural energy) to provide generative power for the dream state. The energy is already *in* the CNS. For D generation there is also no need to postulate the existence of the unconscious as the psychic subsystem or collection of neurons necessary for the storage of the energy of repressed wishes, and there is nothing to suggest that the concept of repression is in any way germane to controlling the activity of the pontine cells responsible for D generation. Intrapontine, autochthonously proceeding, and active cellular mechanisms are all that is required. Further, the concept of regression in the sense of a reversed flow of neural energy is not needed or even correct. The pontine executive cells conduct in the same direction that they do during waking; they just become some 40-fold more active in the D state.

There is also serious difficulty with Freud's theory that the primary motivating force for the dream language and dream plot is disguise of a repressed wish. The driving force for D sleep is a biologically determined and *motivationally neutral* activation of cells in the pons, not a repressed wish. There is no evidence whatsoever that these cellular mechanisms of generation are in any way driven by hunger, sex, or any other instinct or by repressed wishes for consummation of instnctual drives. The *primary motive* for the dream language and dream process cannot be disguised if the prime force of dreams is not an instinct or repressed "wish" in need of disguise.

## After 1960

Dreaming became an electrophysiological phenomenon capable of being recorded. It ceased being a purely subjective human phenomenon and was seen to belong, as Aristotle had guessed, to a large part of the animal kingdom, from birds to (almost all) mammals. It was also detectable in ovo and in utero. Its function as guardian of sleep became difficult to reconcile with that of a *state* as deep as the deepest sleep. What significance is there for a newly hatched chick to realize any desire other than to become a cock or a hen? The whole domain of dream function, apart from a few rear-guard actions, slowly quit the psychoanalyst's couch to enter the neurobiology laboratory. Every one of the numerous research schools of the early 1960s tried to find a function for dreaming to explain neurophysiological mechanisms, phylogenesis, ontogenesis, and the exasperating lack of evidence of problems caused by suppression of dreams, a fact that is often forgotten or hidden.

One should not believe, however, that Freudian dogma on dreams suddenly collapsed. It continued, disillusioned or disguised, but triumphant. Although almost nothing remains of the Freudian model of the "how" of dreaming, it is interesting to summarize briefly the psychoanalysts' concepts of the function of dreams. Their attitudes can be classified into three movements.

### 1.  The Unconditional Supporters of the Freudian Model

We recommend that the reader consult the remarkable article of André Bourguignon.[16] Freudian theory is confronted with the mechanisms of paradoxical sleep. Bourguignon attributes four principle functions to dreams: stimulation, discharge, substitution, and finally liaison. Each of these functions, he claims, has a psychoanalytical explanation and can be substantiated by neurophysiology.

This remarkable research (by modern neurophysiology) neither adds anything important to, nor detracts from, psychoanalysis which, as a theory, can only find new confirmation therein. But this is not surprising for anyone who knows that analytical theory is based on carefully observed facts. The domain of dreaming shows the considerable advance that psychoanalysis has over the biological sciences, to which it has to some extent opened the way ...

## 2.   Those Disillusioned by the Freudian Model

Among these one must cite Charles Fisher. This great physiologist, then psychoanalyst, was a pioneer in studying erection during dreaming (see chapter 8). He can be regarded as one of the founding fathers of the modern neurobiology of dreaming. Fisher concluded an important review article[46] thus:

In most recent theories, the conception of dreaming has become pallid and watered down in comparison to Freud's formulation in terms of the dream as an attempt to deal with those indestructible, especially repressed, unconscious infantile wishes, the mental representations of the great human passions, the instinctual drives. But it must be stated that however important all this has appeared to be when viewed from the chair behind the couch, the experiments reported suggest that human beings seem to be able to function fairly well for prolonged periods of time in the absence of dreaming. Thus, REM sleep and sleep generally become more mysterious the more we learn about them. It may be, as someone has said, "Sleep is to prevent us from wandering around in the dark and bumping into things" (Dement 1972).

## 3.   The Eclectics, or Highjackers of the Freudian Model

The latest avatar of the Freudian theory of the dream as the guardian of sleep is Snyder's view of the dream as a *sentinel*.[147] But for him the dream does not guard an animal's sleep against its repressed desires, but rather against potential enemies.

In all mammals, sleep is a dangerous period because the threshold of arousal is increased. It is, however, interrupted by periods of paradoxical sleep in which cortical electrical activity is similar to that during waking. As Snyder rightly remarks, periods of paradoxical sleep are often followed by fleeting moments of waking before the animal (or man) falls back to sleep. So, if the dream images represented a terrifying scene (such as an attack by predators) this might prepare the individual to face an aggressor (at least through the sympathetic nervous system, if not through the motor system, for there is generalized muscular atonia). Periodic wakening following periods of sleep would be useful to examine the environment briefly for possible predators before falling asleep again. This is the *sentinel hypothesis*. However, in order not to cut himself off entirely from the Freudian world, Snyder insists at the end of his article: "Thus, under conditions of security the hallucinations would be such as to gratify rather than frighten, thus fostering the greater continuity of sleep."

So Snyder drifts imperceptibly, almost remorsefully, from the dream as sentinel to the dream as guardian of sleep. Although he contributed in a remarkable fashion to the objective study of dreaming in chimpanzees and opossums, Snyder cannot shake off his training in psychoanalysis and, in the end, pays homage to the founding father by citing this extract from *The Interpretation of Dreams*: " 'What,' asks the proverb, 'do geese dream of?' and it replies: 'Of maize!!' The whole theory that dreams are wish fulfillments is contained in these two phrases."

Thus Snyder's theory marks a historic stage. It represents a difficult passage, a highjacking of Freudian metaphysics across the border to neurobiology. Later work has shown that there exists a correlation between the quantity of paradoxical sleep and a "security" factor during sleep. But this correlation is the inverse of the one predicted in the sentinel hypothesis. The securer an animal is during sleep, the longer it dreams. (Who wants to attack a sleeping lion, or a ferret in its burrow?) On the other hand, hunted animals, such as herbivores, only have a minute quantity of paradoxical sleep. Why then would the dream sentinel so often be ready to wake animals that sleep securely?

### Paradoxical Sleep, Memory, and Forgetting

Experiments on animals have demonstrated correlations, if not causal relations, between paradoxical sleep and memory.[10,64,65] On the one hand, deprivation of paradoxical sleep can lead to deficits in complex learning processes, and on the other, learning is sometimes followed by a significant increase in paradoxical sleep. In the rat, learning a simple task is not disturbed by deprivation of paradoxical sleep, but if it is complex, deprivation does perturb the task.

According to Greenberg and Pearlman,[58] learning that is acquired rapidly is based on preprogrammed links. This "prepared" learning is not sensitive to deprivation of paradoxical sleep. On the other hand, learning that is acquired slowly is based on nonprogrammed links that require the individual to integrate various forms of unhabitual information and elaborate new behavioral strategies adapted to the situation. This is "unprepared" learning, which can be upset by deprivation of paradoxical sleep.

Carlyle Smith[144,145,146] introduced the concept of "windows" for paradoxical sleep, that is, special periods for paradoxical sleep essential to the acquisition of learning. Smith accumulated data in favor of such windows for the establishment of memories existing for some hours or days after learning. After sessions of task learning the proportion of paradoxical sleep increases consistently, from 30% to 60%. When the task has been fully acquired the duration of paradoxical sleep again becomes identical to that observed in control recordings. This phenomenon of increased paradoxical sleep is seen from the first hour of sleep following the learning session. If animals are deprived of sleep during this first hour after training, the increase in paradoxical sleep no longer happens in subsequent periods of unlimited sleep, and the retention of the learning is severely reduced. But if the deprivation is only imposed after an hour or two of sleep it is without effect on the retention of learning. Thus, the presence of a sufficient quantity of paradoxical sleep in the first hour following learning seems to be a determining factor for stabilizing the memory trace. Here we return to Carlyle Smith's concept of a window for paradoxical sleep.

The interesting findings of Bloch and his colleagues[10] on increased paradoxical sleep after learning raise a number of questions. In particular, they ask if the increase in paradoxical sleep reflects the elaboration of a process of information handling, or if it is merely a consequence of the acquisition itself.

We have known for a long time that the information acquired during a learning session is treated by the brain immediately after the session during a phase of "mnemonic consolidation." We now see that this period must be followed by a minimum amount of paradoxical sleep if there is to be memorization. Thus mnemonic processes involved in the consolidation period and during paradoxical sleep seem closely related, suggesting that they are two critical stages of information handling. It is as if information handling, begun during waking, was taken up again during subsequent paradoxical sleep; the amount of paradoxical sleep needed after the exercise would therefore be a function of the amount of mnemonic information to be handled.[10]

Although there are obviously relationships between para-doxical sleep and learning in animals, one must admit that such relationships have never been demonstrated in man. Adminis-tration of benzodiazepines, which disturb dreaming very little, often cause considerable memory problems, whereas mono-amine oxidase inhibitors, which stop dreaming completely, do not disturb memory.

It seems difficult to accept that sleep plays necessary or essential role in memory. We described a case of total absence of sleep for five days with no memory impairment.[124] We also published the case of a patient with syringomyelia, a painful disease of the spinal cord, who had been prevented from sleeping for more than three months, as verified by continuous polygraph recording.[45] This patient had no problems with memory. There is also the victim of a shrapnel lesion in the pons, described by Lavie,[97] who had no sign of paradoxical sleep for several years. In spite of this, he maintained his pro-fessional activity as a lawyer, which would have been impossi-ble for a person with amnesia.

So I continue to think that the hypothesis that sleeping or dreaming plays an essential role in the transfer of short-term memory to long-term memory is far from proved.

The hypothesis of Crick and Mitchison[27] that we discussed in chapter I is a modern version of Robert's theory of 1886,[133] dressed up with computers and neural networks. Their hypoth-esis can be summarized as follows. The immense complexity of the cerebral cortex can be seen as a neural network. At the heart of this network, information is distributed to an enor-mous number of synapses. Such a network can be overloaded if it has to handle simultaneously models that are too dissimilar or too large. Overloading of the network ought, then, to cause "bizarre" associations, or always reproduce the same associations ("obsessions"). Especially if the network feeds back on itself, it may even respond with "hallucinations" to signals that would normally demand no response. We must therefore be able to eliminate overload, what they called *parasitic modes*, in the network.

The deus ex machina capable of eliminating these parasites might be paradoxical sleep. Dreaming would then be a cleaning process by which the brain, functioning as a closed circuit, could rid itself of all parasitic modes by creating new information circuits stimulated by ponto-geniculo-occipital (PGO) activity. Thus a dream would function as a *reverse learning* mechanism which would modify the cortex, perhaps by altering synaptic transmission. A synapse needs to be "strengthened" in order to remember something; in reverse learning it would be "weakened." Crick and Mitchison thus suggested that during paradoxical sleep we unlearn our subconscious dreams ("We dream in order to forget.") In support of their hypothesis, they cited the theoretical work of John Hopfield and his colleagues,[70] according to which random stimulation of an *artificial* neural network would permit better access to stored memories and would suppress most erroneous ones. So, unlearning could help learning! Of course, Crick and Mitchison did not forget that the prolonged suppression of dreaming (by monoamine oxidase inhibitors) does not cause hallucinations or parasitic thoughts, or memory deficits in man. So they had to admit: "A direct test of our postulated reverse learning mechanism seems extremely difficult ... [One] approach would be to look for the structural and chemical correlates of the postulated reverse learning mechanism, but exactly how to do this is at the moment is unclear. Without further evidence of this kind our theory must be regarded as speculative."

## The Functions of Paradoxical Sleep during Ontogenetic Development

The demonstration of oneiric behavior, the internal game of the brain to use Jean Piaget's excellent metaphor, does not answer the fundamental question, what is the use of paradoxical sleep? Study of ontogenesis could suggest the beginnings of an answer. During paradoxical sleep (or the very similar state of active sleep) there exists an ontogenetic continuity from fetal movements in the rat or guinea pig, to those of newborn rats or kittens (in which the system controlling postural inhibition is not yet completely functional), to those of oneiric behavior in the adult. Fetal movements are probably the expression of maturation in genetically programmed synapses in the central nervous system. Even if we cannot completely exclude the influence of the intrauterine environment on the newborn, it is clear that genetic programming plays a predominant role in determining stereotyped movements of crawling, close contact, and suckling that occur during active sleep in the newborn.

Between 1960 and 1966 study of the ontogenesis of the sleep-wake cycle furnished a rich harvest of surprising data. The more immature a brain at birth, the greater the quantity of active sleep. It can constitute 80% of sleep in a newborn kitten or rat, and 60% in a human neonate. Howard Roffwarg and his colleagues[134] therefore asked what could be the significance of paradoxical sleep just after birth. It could be a passive mechanism due to the absence of control of the immature cerebral cortex over the systems responsible for paradoxical sleep. Or it could be an active mechanism, with active or paradoxical sleep playing a major role in the maturation of the central nervous system during fetal life and later periods of maturation.

The first hypothesis can be abandoned, for removal of the cortex (pathologically in man or experimentally in animals) does not cause increased paradoxical sleep. We must therefore accept that the second hypothesis is the more likely, and try to explain the function of paradoxical sleep in the development of the central nervous system.

Active sleep might provide intense stimulation from endogenous sources at a moment when the organism has little exogenous excitation. Impulses from the brainstem pacemaker might thus contribute to the maturation of thalamocortical pathways. This stimulation might "anticipate" or "prepare" the brain to respond in an appropriate way to future sensory stimulation. We must then explain the persistence of paradoxical sleep in the adult. It must be important as there can be a rebound of paradoxical sleep following its suppression (see chapter 7).

### Is Active Sleep Paradoxical Sleep?

Is there a boundary between active sleep in the fetus, the rat pup, and the kitten, and paradoxical sleep which appears a few weeks after birth with all the characteristics of the adult? Is it the same process? (see chapter 2). Adrien[2] proposed a very important new concept (figure 18):

In precocious species the principal criterion for identifying active sleep is a series of muscle twitches on a background of hypotonia, an activity similar to the phasic phenomena observed during paradoxical sleep, but which do not seem to share the same origin ... These twitches of active sleep could be a reflection of an "intrinsic" property of every motor circuit to trigger suddenly and without central coordination.

Progressively, as the neuronal circuits mature, a supraspinal control system for all these circuits would develop. Active sleep would then be replaced by true "phasic" activity characteristic of paradoxical sleep, originating in a "pontine generator" in the brainstem.

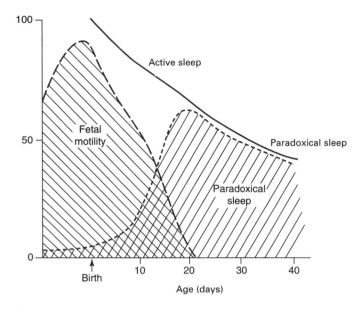

**Figure 18**
Schematic representation of the mechanisms underlying the regulation
of states of vigilance during development. The continuous line is
derived from experimental data obtained in kittens. The dashed lines
represent the possible regulatory mechanisms, and the sum of the two
curves represents the experimental result. The initial embryonic active
sleep is replaced by true paradoxical sleep when the brainstem structures regulating it are sufficiently mature. The progressive replacement
of one mechanism by the other explains the behavioral continuity that
is observed. (From Adrien[2])

It has often been considered that active sleep was an archaic form of
paradoxical sleep, or that the paradoxical sleep of the adult was in some
way the periodic resurgence of a primitive activity. In fact, it would
rather seem that the two behaviors are distinct, with different characteristics, and that they are subject to different forms of regulation.

During development, paradoxical sleep progressively replaces the
active state as the neuronal networks that control it mature. We suggest that figure 3 might represent the behavioral continuity (especially

of phasic motor activity) observed in active and paradoxical sleep during ontogenesis.

## The Programming Hypothesis for Paradoxical Sleep

Edmond Dewan is an information theoretician who derived inspiration from computer programming to propose a model of programming in the brain.[37] In computers you can use two methods to set up a program. Either you connect various components, or you store instructions as numerical codes in the computer's memory. These instructions are then used sequentially. There are two ways of changing the program. Either you replace the instructions in the memory, or utilize a mechanism with intermittent automatic reprogramming. Dewan's hypothesis opted for the second for the brain: its functional structure would be modifiable by spontaneous autoreprogramming. According to him, paradoxical sleep would be adequate for programming.

• It must ensure the initial programming of the embryonic brain, establish new functional circuits after a cerebral lesion and when old neurons die and cannot be replaced (estimated by Dewan at thousands each day, but without giving any evidence!).

• The programming must also play a role in memory processes. As in a computer, some information could be stored in slow-access memories if they are used relatively infrequently. In other cases a faster system must be available. Thus access to information would be more functional.

• Emotion could play a supplementary role in programming. It would be used to "tag" or label memories and programs to consolidate them. Thus, during the programming process "all memories, programs, and so forth that are relevant to a current important need can be brought together and 'filed' in one place by making use of these tags. This is analogous to the computer technique known as 'associative memory' in which the address number of each memory location includes a coded numerical tag to identify the type of information stored there."

Dewan ended his article by proposing some clinical consequences of failure in his programming system, which, like computers, would be subject to breakdown. He suggested that schizophrenia, manic depression, and dyslexia could be explained by a block in the programming system, but did not propose any explanation for the absence of troubles caused by long-term deprivation of dreaming in man.

## Recent Concepts of the Function of Sleep and Paradoxical Sleep

I must acknowledge the exceptional series of studies by Allen Rechtschaffen and his colleagues.[130,131,132] Their experiments, over many years, do not support *a unitary* function for sleep. They rather tend toward a role for sleep in heat regulation, energy conservation, the integrity of the immune system, and tissue repair. Physical sleep deprivation for two or three weeks in rats leads to their death: there is a consistent picture of hypothermia, weight loss, increased metabolic rate, and skin ulcers on the feet and tail, but the precise cause of death remains unclear. It may be that a breakdown of the immune system allows the invasion of lethal opportunistic germs.[40]

We may wonder, however, if the very aggressive technique of sleep deprivation used plays a direct role in these deaths, for we have kept cats in perfect health for more than a month while deprived of slow wave and paradoxical sleep by tiny, localized brain lesions.[138]

I think we are slowly becoming aware that what we call "sleep," with all its different stages, is the expression of complex physiological phenomena, perhaps organized sequentially and perhaps topographically.

We must admit that when we talk of the function of waking we are using a shortcut that means very little. The waking state, however irregular, is a necessary condition for the realization of most vital homeostatic regulation. We need only think of the search for food and its absorption, the search for a sexual partner and mating, the hatching of eggs or suckling of young, the defense of one's territory, and many others. It could be that each of these functions is prepared or regulated during sleep. However, sleep depends of necessity on the external environment.

*The theory of iterative genetic programming* that I propose in the next chapter has been built up from the most recent neurobiological data concerning paradoxical sleep and elements of the theories of Roffwarg, Muzio, Dement, Adrien, and Dewan.

This theory does not entirely resolve the mystery of the functions of dreaming and will doubtless soon seem just as erroneous as all the others that repose in the graveyard of dream theories. It simply reflects the enormous curiosity of an awake brain about dreams.

# 7

# Is Paradoxical Sleep the Guardian of Psychological Individuality?

Genetics has become the science of individuality. It has become interested in the brain. Different behavior in different strains of mice is well-known.[17,66] However, there seems to be resistance in some scientific circles to accepting that there could be a genetic element in explaining psychological differences between individual human beings.[135] Psychological individuality stems from two inextricably linked sources that are difficult to distinguish biologically or experimentally: genetic and epigenetic factors.

One of the best methods to measure the impact of genetic factors is the study of identical and nonidentical twins. The rarity of such observations explains why there have been relatively few publications on this subject. I have already suggested the importance of the work of Tom Bouchard and his colleagues[14,15,68] in chapter 1. They summarized an enormous study of 100 pairs of identical and nonidentical twins since 1979, either brought up together or separated soon after birth and brought up in different environments. These twins were subjected to psychological and physiological tests at the Uni-

Originally published in the *Canadian Journal of Psychology* (1991) 4: 148–168.

versity of Minnesota for a week. The results suggested that about 70% of variation in IQ was genetically determined. Tests of personality, temperament, work and leisure habits, and social attitudes demonstrated a very close similarity between identical twins raised separately and those raised together.

The following example illustrates, in two exceptional cases, the subject of our discussion, that is, genetic determination of psychological individuality. The Jim twins were brought up from early infancy in different families in the American Middle West. They only met 39 years later at the University of Minnesota when they were studied by Bouchard. Their physical and pathological histories were amazingly similar. They both had hemorrhoids. Their heart rates, blood pressure, EEG, and the form of their sleep polygraph recordings were identical. They had both inexplicably put on 5 kg of weight at the same time, and suffered from migraine since the age of 18. Even more astonishing was the story of their affective lives, for they had followed the same route. They had both been divorced from a first wife named Linda, and remarried a wife called Betty. They had both called their dogs Toy and their sons James Allan and James Alan, respectively. The hobby of both was carpentry and both bit their nails.

No one is surprised at the physical resemblance of twins or by characteristic physical traits in certain royal families. The Bourbons' nose is famous. DNA programs and cell division can explain that. It is probably similar for the pathological background of twins, for they possess the same enzymes and metabolic errors. But how do you explain their psychological heredity, responsible for identical idiosyncratic behavior in twins exposed to different environments all their life?

Must we accept that the genetic program of pre- and post-natal development must suffice, *once and for all*, for the innumerable subtle interneuronal connections that will be responsible for a given character trait for the whole of a lifetime? Such a hypothesis is improbable. On the one hand, the genetic programming of thousands of billions of synaptic connections would necessitate far more genes than exist in the genome. On the other hand, environmental influences would in any case alter these connections in the end, for neurons are endowed with extraordinary plasticity, as I have emphasized several times already. Thus, exposing a fetal rat to certain drugs or hormones can modify its behavior throughout its life.[19] Rearing mice in the dark can alter definitively the structure of the visual cortex,[71] and suturing closed the eyelids of a kitten disconnects the afferents to the visual cortex and modifies cortical electrical activity and the branching pattern of nerve fibers in the visual cortex.[156] Sensory deprivation or exposure to an "enriched" environment can also alter the cellular and enzymatic architecture of the cortex.[59] The list of anatomical and biochemical modifications in the brain caused by the internal or external environment grows daily and it has become obvious that neuronal connections can be modified by experience. How, then, can we explain the conservation of certain personality traits in twins subjected for several decades since birth to different experiences that leave their different imprints on their nervous systems?

If we accept the existence of genetic factors in the organization of behavioral patterns, it seems difficult to understand how a genetic program, established *definitively* by the end of maturation, could remain effective in organizing psychological individuation in spite of modifications produced by the environment through the process of synaptic plasticity. For these reasons, the concept of periodic or "iterative" genetic "reprogramming" seems more satisfactory. This endogenous process would excite at regular intervals the synaptic structures responsible for psychological individuation.

## Neurogenesis

During ontogenesis, neurogenesis is the guardian of individuality through its contribution to the genetically programmed organization of the central nervous system. If neurons continued to divide throughout adult life (*continuous neurogenesis*), like most cells in the body, we could imagine that their DNA program could transmit an identical hereditary psychological patrimony to each twin. However, neurons of the central nervous system do not divide, with few exceptions.

In cold-blooded fish, amphibians, and reptiles, the brain continues to grow throughout life, with continuous neurogenesis.[69] For example, in fish there is continuous replacement of certain olfactory neurons whose axons project to central neurons. Continuous neurogenesis contributes to keeping "imprinted" information throughout life, explaining, for example, the homing behavior of salmon.[62] In amphibians, continuous neurogenesis exists in the visual pathways, and in lizards postnatal neurogenesis has been described in the cerebral cortex.[101] There also seems to be a correlation between the existence of continuous neurogenesis and the capacity for regeneration in the central nervous system, for in some fish the caudal part of the spinal cord can be entirely reconstituted after sectioning.[69]

The appearance of warm-bloodedness, permitting greater freedom in relation to the temperature of the environment, was accompanied by a considerable reduction in capacity for postnatal neurogenesis.

Birds seem to represent a transitional stage: their brain has many similarities to that of fish, amphibians, and reptiles.[92] New neurons can appear in the forebrain of adult birds. In some cases new neurons can be incorporated in functional circuits, for example, the system responsible for song in canaries and zebra finches.[116,122] It seems that this process for adult neurogenesis appears seasonally, under the influence of sex steroids.

In contrast, these phenomena do not exist in mammals, in which neurogenesis disappears within a month of birth (indeed in humans it is essentially finished by midgestation). Instead of neurogenesis there is actual regression, with death of cell bodies and retraction of axons during adult life. This regression is accompanied by a considerable decrease in the capacity of central neurons to regenerate.[42,120]

So the preservation of genetic individuality through continuous neurogenesis in the adult seems possible in cold-blooded animals. It is also possible, but seasonal, in some adult birds. It is virtually impossible in postnatal mammals. The mechanism that gave the Bourbons their nose is therefore absent from mammalian neurons.

We must suppose that a new mode of genetic programming appeared together with warm-bloodedness. Learning necessitates constant repetition of epigenetic stimuli in order to establish the morphological and biochemical bases of new neuronal connections. So why not conceive that certain genetic programs may be reinforced periodically (*iterative* programming) in order to establish and maintain the function of synaptic circuits responsible for psychological heredity? This mechanism could thus interact with the environment by *reestablishing* certain circuits that have been altered by epigenetic factors and, conversely, by *suppressing* others.

### Can Paradoxical Sleep Program the Individuality of the Central Nervous System?

Probably as an admission of ignorance, I now return to a personal hypothesis that I proposed in chapter 1. It is unchallengeable and therefore nonscientific. My thesis is that our dreams make each of us different because during them a repetitive program wipes out certain aspects of what we have learned, and may reinforce others if they are compatible with the "genetic program" of the dream.

I shall review the experimental facts that support the hypothesis that genetic programming of the brain occurs during paradoxical sleep. To facilitate the discussion I shall also summarize a theoretical model of genetic programming of the brain. This model presupposes a synchronic (internal) organization. It equally presupposes a diachronic temporal organization, related to the history of the individual, that is, to epigenetic events. It is developed from our published hypotheses,[78,80,82] elaborated thanks to the commentaries of Claude Debru.[29]

There seems to be an inverse relationship between neurogenesis and paradoxical sleep during both phylogeny and ontogeny.

1. There is no paradoxical sleep in cold-blooded animals, in which neurogenesis can guarantee genetic programming of the brain throughout life using classic DNA mechanisms in dividing immature neurons. (Paradoxical sleep exists in most mammals, but not in dolphins as we have seen, nor in monotremes—the duck-billed platypus and the echidna—although their slow wave sleep is accompanied by relative hypothermia. It would be of the greatest interest to discover if continuous neurogenesis exists in these species.)

2. Episodes of paradoxical sleep are very brief (about ten seconds) in birds in which adult neurogenesis is possible.
3. Paradoxical sleep gradually supersedes active sleep as neurogenesis disappears during postnatal development of mammals.

So the question remains: can paradoxical sleep renew genetic programming in species in which neurogenesis ends at the end of ontogenesis?

## Does Psychological Heredity Need Repeated Genetic Programming?

The respective importance of heredity and the environment (nature and nurture) in determining personality is one of the domains of psychology that has given rise to the most animated debates. This has been calculated theoretically,[69] and Bouchard's results,[14,15] described above, on identical twins brought up from birth in totally different environments leave little doubt about the existence of psychological heredity.

Iterative programming of the brain during paradoxical sleep would reinforce or obliterate the traces of epigenetic learning occurring during waking.[82] Periodic dreaming would permit the repeated programming of unconscious reactions that are the basis of personality and individual differences in behavior in subjects exposed to the same environments.

A genetic program implies selection associated with non-predictive (Epimethean) evolution. So, there exists in a population of mice, for example, enough polymorphism to produce aggressive or timid individuals, some slow to learn, others fast, some inhibited by emotion, others not. Thus some individuals will survive, perhaps the aggressive ones or the timid ones, according to the laws of natural selection. Can we extrapolate and speak of a hereditary potential to be timid or aggressive, musician or mathematician, if the environment permits it or at least does not prevent it?

As guardians and intermittent programmers of the hereditary part of our personality, it is possible that dreams also play a less conservational, predictive (Promethean) role.[118] Indeed, thanks to the extraordinary diversity of possible connections in our brain as the basic circuits of our personality are programmed, an infinitely variable set of permutations could emerge—influenced ~~by acquired~~ by acquired experience—engendering the fantasies that make up dreams, or preparing new thought structures that will enable us to tackle new problems.

So we can easily conceive the importance of the hundred minutes of dreaming that occur periodically every night, when our body temperature is at its lowest. These hundred minutes of dreaming, of which we can neither trigger the start nor control the contents, certainly play a major role in the first few years of life. They probably continue to repeatedly program the subtlest reactions of our waking consciousness. Rimbaud's poetic genius already remarked: "I am another."

### Iterative Programming

The programming of circuits responsible for hereditary idiosyncrasies does not need the production of new neurons by neurogenesis. Existing cell bodies contain the necessary DNA for the synthesis of proteins to be incorporated in membranes as receptors. So I propose that certain types of neuron that appear late in ontogenesis, such as some interneurons,[73] can synthesize receptors continuously. Such "labile" receptors would only become functional if they were "stabilized" by endogenous excitation. We must therefore assume the existence of an *endogenous generator* that would be responsible for the "validation" of these receptors, just as epigenetic stimuli maintain function in the visual pathway. There is no need for temporal coding of impulses from the generator in order to "instruct" this validation (my "instructive" hypothesis[78]). According to a simpler "selective" hypothesis,[80,82] information for the hereditary program would depend only on the selection of neurons that are, or are not, excited by a randomly coded endogenous program. According to this selective hypothesis a limited number of genes could contribute to the programming of psychological heredity by inducing the synthesis of receptors and ensuring the presence of presynaptic terminals from the generator in different groups of neurons (figure 19).

There are still no direct data concerning the possible synthesis of receptors before paradoxical sleep and their "stabilization" during it. Some results indirectly support the existence of protein synthesis dependent on paradoxical sleep. On the one hand a high-molecular-weight protein appears in the brain when paradoxical sleep is reestablished after injection of serotonin in an animal deprived of sleep by an injection of parachlorophenylalanine.[11] On the other hand, an inhibitor of protein synthesis, chloramphenicol, has a powerful inhibitory action on paradoxical sleep. At high doses it suppresses it,[125] while at low doses it causes an *uncoupling* between PGO activity and postsynaptic electrical responses in many parts of the brain.[38] As chloramphenicol can inhibit the synthesis of postsynaptic receptors,[127] it seems possible that the uncoupling may be due to inhibition of synthesis of genetically programmed receptors on target cells. In this case PGO activity could longer excite neural systems via interneurons. It would be no more than insignificant "noise" invading a brain deprived of receptors capable of making it function: an *empty dream*.

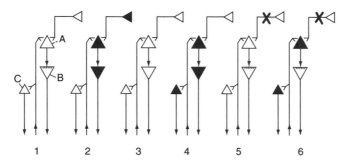

**Figure 19**
Theoretical model of iterative genetic programming during paradoxical sleep. 1. An interneuron (B) has synthesized a labile membrane receptor (vertical hatching). 2. During paradoxical sleep the PGO system (upper right) stimulates interneuron A, which excites and "stabilizes" the receptor of neuron B, and makes it functional. 3. This receptor remains functional during the period of waking that follows paradoxical sleep. 4. As long as the receptor is functional, environmental stimuli (ascending arrow) can activate both nonspecific arousal responses (system C) and the idiosyncratic genetically programmed response from B. 5. If paradoxical sleep is suppressed and there is no more PGO activity, the receptor remains labile and nonfunctional and neuron B is no longer activated. 6. In this case the epigenetic stimulus will no longer be able to trigger idiosyncratic responses, but only nonspecific ones. (From Jouvet[80])

This recurrent programming, which we might call *endogenous phylogenetic learning*, could theoretically be envisaged in two forms (figure 20). In the first, the *presynaptic* influence of PGO activity would be responsible for the programming. The arrival of PGO information as electrical impulses along axons would in some way modify the synaptic receptors by a mechanism analogous to that of environmental stimuli during waking. This hypothesis is not very plausible for it is difficult to imagine how a receptor could be modified by PGO activity to code such an enormous amount of information.

Presynaptic mechanism

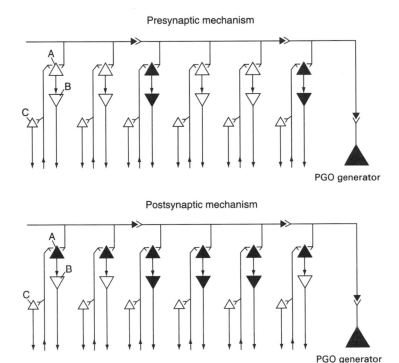

PGO generator

Postsynaptic mechanism

PGO generator

**Figure 20**
Hypothetical programming mechanisms. In the presynaptic programming mechanism (top) the patterns of PGO activity are coded. This information from the PGO generator is transmitted through a polysynaptic pathway to different interneurons. Some recognize this message and are selectively programmed. According to this theory we must assume that at the generator proteins are responsible for a spatiotemporal coding capable of programming the different interneurons successively. In the postsynaptic programming mechanism (bottom) PGO activity is less rigidly genetically determined, and has no programming effect. It triggers all interneurons. There is then a selection of postsynaptic targets according to the cycle of synthesis of postsynaptic receptors (see figure 19). The second mechanism is the more plausible. It explains the selective firing of interneurons in relation to PGO activity during paradoxical sleep, as demonstrated by Steriade.[148]

This is why the hypothesis of *postsynaptic* coding seems more likely. In this case, neurons involved in handling phylogenetically important stimuli would continually synthesize receptors. These receptors would then be "validated" by the PGO information, enabling them to function as a response to epigenetic trigger stimuli. The release of stereotyped oneiric behavior at the same time as the stimulation and validation of these receptors could then be regarded as endogenous phylogenetic learning. This mechanism would help explain the numerous cases of an apparent predisposition to learning, in that an animal learns complex behavior immediately as long as the trigger signal is phylogenetically important.

## Mechanisms and Theoretical Conditions for Iterative Genetic Programming

The endogenous generator must be able to act on both sensory systems and cortical and subcortical motor systems. In the former case it might induce irrelevant percepts, or hallucinations. In the latter it might maintain or facilitate programs responsible for individual idiosyncratic behavior, or even suppress or alter other learned motor programs. It thus seems that programmed excitation must be able to act directly on brainstem or spinal cord motor neurons.

As motor neurons would be subject to the influence of endogenous programming, there should be two consequences:

1. It should be possible to distinguish a genetic component in the patterns of activity of motor neurons that are directly or indirectly controlled by the generator during programming. This genetic component would be due to the triggering of different groups of motor neurons in response to random excitation by the endogenous generator.

2. There should equally exist mechanisms to suppress muscle activity during motor or sensory programming, without which the organism might be subject to hallucinations or uncontrolled stereotyped motor behavior, which could be dangerous, whether it happened during waking or sleep.

In order for genetic programming to take place without too much "background noise," that is, with a high signal-to-noise ratio, there must also be control mechanisms to inhibit the arrival of internal or external sensory stimuli. In this way integrative processes would be facilitated, just as happens during attentiveness in waking life. The brain would neither receive nor respond to external (and probably some internal) stimuli at the moment of genetic programming, as a result of inhibition of sensory input and the blocking of muscle activity. Therefore, *a protective* mechanism should exist to allow this process to appear only when the organism is not subject to potentially dangerous stimuli, that is, when arousal mechanisms are no longer active, *which means during sleep.*

A raised sensory threshold is a well-known phenomenon when paying attention to something (or being distracted) during waking, and also during paradoxical sleep. It disappears during slow wave sleep. It corresponds to a decrease in cortical or thalamic evoked responses in the somatosensory, auditory, and visual systems.[126] It is therefore probable that this centrifugal control is responsible for the great increase in the threshold for arousal during paradoxical sleep, but its precise mechanism is unknown. It is therefore impossible to verify the hypothesis of signal-to-noise ratio that we mentioned earlier. For example, does the suppression of centrifugal control modify the secondary process of PGO activity and its expression in oneiric behavior?

## Synchronic Aspects of Programming

The *patterns* of PGO activity defy classification, although Chouvet[24] proposed a model for the cat. It is not possible to discuss in detail here the difficulties and the results of these analyses. Very briefly, the "coding" of PGO activity seems to consist of two different processes. The primary process might represent the spontaneous activity of the pontine generator. The secondary process might reflect the response of interneurons in the oculomotor system and already contain part of the expression of the genetic programming, for it is dependent on the primary process. It is in fact possible to considerably modify the patterns of PGO activity during paradoxical sleep by decortication.[75]

For this reason it is easier to study synchronic aspects of programming at the effector organs, triggered by the genetically programmed receptors excited by the primary random process. This is only possible by using eye movements, which are not inhibited during paradoxical sleep. Results obtained in mice from two genetically "pure" strains (BALB/c and C57BR/cd) reveal very different patterns, while analysis in breeding experiments of hybrids of the first generation and backcrosses confirms the existence of genetic dominance in the C57BR/cd strain.[21,24] Bert also described a different organization of patterns of PGO activity in two species of baboon (*Papio papio* and *Papio hamadryas*).[9] Finally, Chouvet et al.[25] observed considerable individual variation in the temporal organization of eye movements during paradoxical sleep in ten unrelated young adult men, while the organization was similar in six pairs of identical twins. In summary, the results of analysis of eye movements during paradoxical sleep in genetically pure strains of mice and in young identical human twins support a genetic component.

However, patterns of eye movements do not enable us to determine the type of behavior that is programmed during paradoxical sleep. That is why we began to study other motor responses that are normally inhibited in paradoxical sleep. We can destroy the systems responsible for motor inhibition during paradoxical sleep in the cat, and so see motor activity resulting from programming during paradoxical sleep by revealing it externally as oneiric behavior (see chapter 4).

Ethnological analysis of oneiric behavior has not enabled us to distinguish typical or invariable stereotyped behavioral patterns. *Each animal has its own repertoire.* One cat may always demonstrate 60% of aggressive behavior, whereas in another such behavior may be almost absent and grooming will dominate. Hunger or thirst does not change the amounts of aggressive or drinking behavior.

It is very likely that PGO activity is the basis for this behavior because it is always present, in its primary and secondary forms, but its complexity has always prevented us from correlating it with different repertoires. Low doses of chloramphenicol reduce stereotyped oneiric behavior considerably.[4] The cat remains motionless, trapped in paradoxical sleep without dreams, while PGO activity is made up almost exclusively of primary processes, and the electrical activity of the brainstem, resulting from excitation of postsynaptic receptors, decreases markedly.

It is not possible to carry out genetic experiments on behavior in cats, so we must await success in obtaining oneiric behavior in different genetically pure strains of mice. Then we shall be able to note any differences in behavior between strains and the distribution of different patterns in different hybrids and backcrosses. Thus we may be able to determine which chromo-some carries the gene or genes that select the targets for PGO activity.

## Diachronic Modalities of Iterative Programming

Genetic programming is obviously predominant during onto-genesis, that is, during the period of organization of the central nervous system by neurogenesis in utero or in ovo. Afterward, the duration of programming can only decrease, if it can only happen during sleep. We might therefore suppose that in the adult a relationship should exist between the duration of pro-gramming and that of sleep.

We must suppose that programming of the central nervous system needs a large quantity of energy, at least equal to that used during learning while awake. Energy reserves are accu-mulated during sleep as glycogen[57,89] which could provide the energy necessary for programming. The best solution would therefore be to devise a periodic functioning, each period of programming being followed by a period of renewal of reserves during sleep. Thus iterative programming would take place in a periodic fashion.

In order to be effective, periodic genetic programming must be related to epigenetic stimuli that have excited the central nervous system during the preceding period of waking. This implies that mechanisms should exist to adapt the duration of programming to the amount of external or internal stimulation that has induced epigenetic modification in systems influenced by the synapses being programmed.

However, genetic programming of personality is indifferent to the destiny of the individual. It is *a law* and has no reason to facilitate the imprinting of the events that have excited the brain. Doubtless, in some cases, programming might facilitate learning by reinforcing certain idiosyncratic personality traits. In other cases, it should have no effect, or even may inhibit or erase certain epigenetically developed synaptic circuits, if they are contrary to typology. This concept of the erasure of certain cortical circuits during paradoxical sleep[80] was particularly developed by Crick and Mitchison.[27] According to them, as we saw in chapter 6, one function of paradoxical sleep would be to unlearn certain undesirable "parasitic modes" in the cortex. Their postulated process of "reverse learning" could serve to forget: "We dream in order to forget." Thus, the suppression of genetic programming might inhibit, facilitate, or have no effect on learning. In contrast, we should expect that such suppression might alter the expression of idiosyncratic behavior and so decrease variance between individuals belonging to different genetic strains within the same species.

Although many other hypotheses are possible,[110] the evolution of paradoxical sleep during phylogenesis could support the hypothesis that this state might represent the acquisition of a new mechanism of individualization when continuous neurogenesis disappeared.

## Deprivation of Paradoxical Sleep and Its Paradoxes

One of the first methods used to determine the function or functions of paradoxical sleep was to attempt to suppress it physically.[32] These experiments uncovered a "rebound" phenomenon. They did not, however, reveal specific alterations of behavior that could be definitely attributed to the absence of paradoxical sleep.

Physical deprivation of paradoxical sleep (using a swimming pool for rats and cats, or waking a human subject as soon as the first signs of paradoxical sleep appear) is followed by well-defined phenomena. On the one hand there is a need to catch up on paradoxical sleep, manifested by its more and more frequent appearance, with episodes almost every minute after deprivation for twenty-four hours in a cat. On the other hand, there is *rebound*, that is, an increase in the relative amount of paradoxical sleep after the end of the deprivation period. The duration of the rebound is proportional to the duration of the deprivation and tends to "repay" in part (50% to 80%) the paradoxical sleep "debt."

This rebound phenomenon was initially explained by a hypothesis of accumulation of "oneirogenic" factors during deprivation. They would be responsible for an increased pressure for paradoxical sleep, before being used up during the rebound.[33,81] This hypothesis led to a search in the brain, or in the cerebrospinal fluid, for oneirogenic peptides. In spite of numerous factors that increase sleep, no specific factor acting on paradoxical sleep has been isolated so far.[12]

Another hypothesis seems more likely to explain paradoxical sleep rebound. It would not be due to the suppression of paradoxical sleep but to the stress of the deprivation releasing pituitary or hypothalamic factors. The experimental evidence is as follows:

• Physical or pharmacological deprivation of paradoxical sleep is not followed by rebound in some strains of mice, such as BALB/c.[90]

• Deprivation of paradoxical sleep by "nonaggressive" methods, such as stroking a cat at the start of each episode, is not followed by rebound.[119]

• The stress of immobilizing a rat for two hours is followed by a large increase in paradoxical sleep.[129]

• The elimination of stress systems suppresses rebound. This has been shown in two ways. Lesions in the arcuate nucleus of the hypothalamus plus removal of the pituitary gland suppress paradoxical sleep rebound in rats.[158] Deprivation of paradoxical sleep by electroshock in a "pontine" cat (with the pituitary and hypothalamus disconnected from the brainstem) is never followed by rebound.[75]

Thus it is very likely that only physical situations capable of causing a particular form of stress can cause rebound. It would be induced either by the intermediary of factors from the arcuate nucleus—for example, peptides[23]—or directly or indirectly by still unknown pituitary factors.

We suppose that the stress of physical deprivation of paradoxical sleep would induce major changes in the cerebral cortex which, in turn, could release pituitary or hypothalamic mechanisms of stress. Indeed, it has been demonstrated that "neuronal stress" (white noise or flashes of light) does not cause the release of hypothalamo-pituitary stress factors if the related cortical sensory area has been removed.[44] It thus seems possible that paradoxical sleep rebound is a mechanism to reestablish cortical circuits altered by various constraints imposed on the organism.

## The Paradox of the Absence of Effects of Deprivation of Paradoxical Sleep in Humans

It is obviously not ethical to suppress paradoxical sleep pharmacologically in a twin to try to detect alterations in psychological individuality compared with the untreated identical control. This is probably why there are relatively few long-term paradoxical sleep deprivation studies in humans. So we have not been able to recognize specific syndromes related to such derivation. Hundreds, if not thousands, of patients with narcolepsy or depression have been treated for periods of months by monoamine oxidase inhibitors or tricyclic antidepressants. These drugs totally, or almost totally, suppress paradoxical sleep, as proved by numerous polygraph recordings during sleep.[46] No memory deficits have been detected, but there are certainly changes in temperament and personality in these subjects. However, because they are depressed it is difficult to attribute this solely to deprivation of paradoxical sleep.

### Learning and Paradoxical Sleep

The literature on the effect of deprivation of paradoxical sleep on learning contains similar numbers of positive and negative results.[153] A relative increase in paradoxical sleep in certain strains of mice immediately after learning is an established fact,[64,102,146] but the effects of its suppression also seem to depend essentially on the strain studied—and thus on its genetic program. The following example is particularly instructive.[91] The strains C57BR and C57BL/6 have the same genetic origin (the C57 strain). They demonstrate the same circadian patterns for slow wave sleep and paradoxical sleep, and have the same total amount of sleep. Each "repays" 60% of its paradoxical sleep "debt" after physical or pharmacological deprivation. However, each strain has different behavior. C57BR mice are more active when running freely and "learn" more quickly in a Y-shaped maze. Thus, after three daily sessions of fifteen trials, 70% of C57BR mice avoid shocks when they mark mistakes, while only 15% of C57BL/6 mice do so. The phenotypic difference between the two strains is thus 55%. If paradoxical sleep is suppressed for ten hours after each session, either physically of pharmacologically, retention of learning is reduced to 60% in the C57BR mice on the third day, while it is increased to 45% in the C57BL/6 mice. There is therefore a difference of only 15%. What is more, whereas deprivation of paradoxical sleep for ten hours has no effect on free-running spontaneous activity in the C57BR mice (from 86% to 82%), it increases spontaneous activity in the C57BL/6 mice from 65% to 89%. So phenotypic variation of spontaneous activity or learning can be considerably reduced by suppression of paradoxical sleep (see above).

These results do not, of course, prove that paradoxical sleep is responsible for iterative genetic programming and for the phenotypic variation between the two C57 strains (in which each individual is a copy of the others), for paradoxical sleep deprivation can act on other processes. However, such results permit us to suppose that it is illusory to test the effects of deprivation of paradoxical sleep on a genetically heterogeneous population, because each individual can act differently.

## "Instinctive Behavior" and Paradoxical Sleep

In 1978 I formulated the hypothesis that paradoxical sleep could contribute to programming species-specific instinctive behavior[78] (see also chapter 4). Oneiric behavior in the cat resembles normal stereotyped behavior of cats, such as stalking, attack, and flight. Thus aimless oneiric behavior is similar to play. This seems to confirm Piaget's hypothesis according to which dreaming is like an intrinsic game of the brain. However, this hypothesis does not seems plausible to me for the following reasons:

1. Instinctive behavior of the newborn, such as searching for the nipple and sucking, would seem to be the only instinctive behavior in humans. Its program must depend essentially on

structural organization imposed by neurogenesis in the brain. It cannot need iterative programming, because in immature neonates it precedes the appearance of true paradoxical sleep (see above).

2. One need only watch kittens playing to see that their waking games are quite adequate to adapt them progressively and perfect their stalking, attack, and flight behavior. Why, then, would dream play be necessary while there is waking play?

3. The very great variability in the repertory of oneiric behavior from one animal to another, and its consistency in an individual animal, forces us to conclude that it is not the typological behavior of the species that is programmed, but on the contrary its phenotypic variability.

4. Finally, Monique Olivo demonstrated in a thesis that physical or pharmacological suppression of paradoxical sleep is incapable of suppressing the maternal behavior in prepubertal, virgin rats that can be triggered by presenting them with newborn pups.

### Evolution and Paradoxical Sleep

One of the essential concepts of evolution is a formal acceptance of intraspecific individual variability, as opposed to a typological conception of the species. This variability can easily be explained by genetic control of somatic characteristics. So why not consider it at the level of psychological processes, as Mayr[108] did?

Genetic variability is universal, a fact which is significant not only for the student of morphology but also for the student of behavior. It is not only wrong to speak of the monkey, but even of the rhesus monkey ... The time has come to stress the existence of genetic differences in behavior ... Striking differences have been described for predator-prey relations, for the reactions of birds to mimicking or to warning colorations, for child care among primates, and for maternal behavior in rats. It is generally agreed by observers that much of this individual difference is not affected by experience but remains essentially constant throughout the entire lifetime of the individual. Such variability is of the greatest interest to the student of evolution, and it is to be hoped that it will receive more attention from the experimental psychologist than it has in the past.

## Conclusion

The theory that I have discussed in this chapter is the response of a neurophysiologist to Mayr's desire, expressed at the time that paradoxical sleep, that enigma of brain function, was discovered.

When I proposed the theory that the probable function of paradoxical sleep was to preserve individuality, I never involved the word "dream." The hypothesis of repetitive genetic programming during paradoxical sleep in no way predicts the presence of dream activity. Of course, it should be possible to detect certain "psychological patterns" related to the personality of dreamers during a long series of dream studies. For instance, subjects programmed to be introverted or aggressive should have series of dreams relating to that aspect of their personality.

It would certainly be interesting to collect long series of dreams in identical twins living in different environments, but that is not easy! In any case, even when I have been able to find evidence for identical dream recall in identical twins who have lived together, I do not believe this proves my theory.

# 8

## Forty Years of Dream Research, or The Collapse of Paradigms

One evening in April 1970, at the end of the annual conference of the Association for Psychophysiological Study of Sleep (APSS) in Santa Fe, New Mexico, I had occasion to participate in a meeting with a dozen or so friends who since 1960 had been involved in research on the mechanisms of sleep and dreams. The aim of the informal meeting was to reflect on the achievements of our research during the decade from 1960 to 1970 and to try a few predictions for 1970 to 1990.

### First, the Balance

The 1960s had been particularly rich: a third state of brain function had been described, probably corresponding to dream activity.

Dreaming had thus become a physiological process and we thought that neurophysiological methods would enable us to resolve the mystery of its mechanisms and therefore of its function or functions.

We already knew where in the brainstem the machinery for dreaming was located and we supposed that electrophysiology would allow us to understand how that machinery was involved in exciting the cerebral cortex periodically during sleep.

The major outline of the ontogenetic and phylogenetic evolution of paradoxical sleep had just been completed. The dolphin and the duck-billed platypus were mysteries because they did not dream, but this trick of Nature did not disturb the order that we perceived through evolution. Dreaming appeared with the birds and the mammals, or in other words, with warm-bloodedness.

Neuropharmacology, aided by the recent development of psychopharmacology, had taught us that it was possible to selectively suppress dreaming with new molecules, such as monoamine oxidase inhibitors. Thus the doorway to brain monoamines (catecholamines and serotonin) was half open, perhaps offering us a way of resolving the mystery of the alternation of the three states of the brain: waking, sleeping, and dreaming. Several of us were asking whether the catecholamines could be responsible for waking and dreaming, and serotonin for sleep. "Wet" neurophysiology (the study of neurotransmitters) was probably set to win the day against the old "dry" neurophysiology (electrophysiology).

Experiments on deprivation of paradoxical sleep (or of dreams in man) had demonstrated a rebound of paradoxical sleep of which the intensity was a function of the duration of the deprivation. There seemed to be a "debt" on the one hand and a "repayment" on the other, while the intensity of the rebound gave birth to the metaphor of "REM pressure."

At the end of the 1960s two concepts had emerged. Paradoxical sleep or dreaming must have an important function because of this compensation if it was suppressed. Unfortunately, even if it was important, we still did not understand it! Some proposed a "hydraulic" model of paradoxical sleep deprivation, which implied the accumulation of an "oneirogenic" factor in the cerebrospinal fluid. The increase of this "REM juice," as my friend William Dement called it, would be responsible for the rebound. We adopted the same hydraulic model that Freud and Lorenz used to explain pulsions. This was the ontogenesis of dream theory, but it retarded the evolution of the discipline.

## The Predictions for 1990

Probably due in part to a certain euphoria resulting from the immoderate consumption of whisky or gin, we agreed on the following predictions for 1990.

Most of us thought that the mechanisms and functions of sleep would be elucidated. We also agreed that the mechanisms of the periodic triggering of dreaming would be known and oneirogenic factors identified. In contrast, none of us thought that we would manage to explain dream imagery or waking consciousness in neuronal terms. Knowledge of the mechanisms of paradoxical sleep ought to enable us to discover its function or functions or, for some, its total absence of function! Finally, we would have discovered drugs enabling us to either induce physiological sleep or prolong it, and to produce good-quality waking periods lasting several days. In the last case these drugs had to be different from amphetamines in that they would cause neither tolerance nor dependence.

Twenty years later we were only seven, and were still friends. Our society had changed its name but not its abbreviation (APSS). It was now called the Association of Professional Sleep Societies. What about our predictions?

The mechanisms of sleep remained obscure, even if we now understood how brain waves become synchronized or slower as sleep deepens.

We were beginning to understand how the internal circadian clock in the hypothalamus controls our waking and sleeping thanks to factors in the cerebrospinal fluid.

But we were still ignorant of why we sleep, even though we glimpsed that we might have to look at the level of brain energy mechanisms.

The mechanisms of the executive systems of paradoxical sleep (that is, the neuronal orchestras that play oneiric melodies under the influence of the invisible PGO conductor) were better known. We even knew "how" some systems worked. For example, since 1958 we had known that paradoxical sleep is accompanied by almost complete atonia. This was attributed to the action of the inhibitory reticular formation, so in vogue at that time. Gradually the anatomical levels of this system were uncovered: the pontine command level, the pontomedullary pathway, the descending spinal system (see chapter 2).

What about the periodic mechanism, the ultradian clock or pacemaker of dreams? Progress was much slower on this. The periodicity of the pacemaker is closely related to the weight of the animal, the weight of its brain, and its metabolism. So the periodicity of a mouse is ten minutes, of a cat 25 minutes, of a man 90 minutes, and of an elephant 180 minutes. "All very well," reply the skeptics, "but it is the same for heart rate and breathing!" However, we discovered how to vary the pacemaker, which was formerly considered as being invariably linked to the species. We saw how it can be regulated by peptides that can speed it up or slow it down. We could also influence it by varying certain aspects of energy regulation in the brain. And we suspected that there could be multiple pacemakers. Perhaps if we ultimately learn all the "hows" about the ultradian pacemakers, it will teach us part of the "why," but we are not yet there.

And what about the oneirogenic factor, the REM juice predicted by the hydraulic model of paradoxical sleep rebound?
First we found one (VIP, or vasoactive intestinal polypeptide),
then two. Now there are ten, or maybe more. We might as well
say that there are none, and that the hydraulic model was a
trap. The rebound of paradoxical sleep after its deprivation is,
indeed, not provoked by an increase in a hypothetical oneiri-
genic factor but by numerous hypothalamo-pituitary factors
released by the stress of the deprivation (see chapter 7). So any
stressful event in our waking life can unleash a cascade of
events, by a mechanism that we are now beginning to understand, which increases the duration of the first dreams of the
night as we fall asleep.

So, had we found a function for dreaming or paradoxical
sleep in 1990? The answer is no, but not because of a lack of
hypotheses. During the previous twenty years we had learned
to handle drugs aimed at treating hypersomnia, especially narcolepsy, and depression. Most of these drugs (monoamine oxidase inhibitors and tricyclics) completely suppress dreaming,
both subjectively and objectively, as judged by sleep recordings. However, some subjects can lead a completely normal
life, with no deficit in memory, for weeks or months in spite of
total suppression of paradoxical sleep.

Pharmacologists have not yet discovered drugs allowing us
to induce or prolong physiological sleep. Of course it is easy to
fall asleep quickly by taking benzodiazepines, but they lead to
tolerance, then dependence, then insomnia as soon as they are
stopped. In twenty years important progress had only been
made in aspects of waking. The discovery of what I call eugre-
goric drugs (such as the new nonamphetamine compound
modafinil) that allow high-quality waking (G. *eu*, good +
*egeirein*, to awaken) has enabled us to abandon amphetamines

in the treatment of most hypersomnia. I used modafinil for more than ten years in the treatment of narcolepsy. These drugs cause neither tolerance nor dependence, and a better knowledge of their mechanism of action should soon endow us with a better knowledge of the mechanisms of arousal.

So, on the whole, in 1990 we were a long way from attaining the objectives we set in 1970. It is very easy to understand why a posteriori. The set of aims that we proposed in 1970, like all attempts at predicting the future, had little chance of success. There is no way of telling what will happen in a few months or years when dealing with complex systems. That is why, politically, economically, and scientifically, those who predict the future later have the greatest difficulty explaining why things did not happen as they had promised!

### The Evolution of Sleep Research and Major Achievements in the Last Decade

One might wonder what has happened since 1990. There have been few major discoveries to change the face of hypno-oneirology, of the type that made the headlines in scientific journals or newspapers. There have been some constructive and some destructive processes which modified our learning curve about dreaming, which was looking promising during the 1960s.

Neuroscience has followed the exponential development of molecular biology, but twenty years late. In 1970 we knew of five or six "respectable" neurotransmitters capable of explaining the "integrative" function of the brain. Now there are about a hundred, of which fifteen or so represent the "jet set" of transmitters.

New, ever more sophisticated techniques have arrived. Since 1983 we can inactivate or stimulate just the cell body of neurons. All the results of experiments carried out before 1983 using electrolytic lesions, which destroy not only the cell bodies but also axons passing through the lesioned area, are now looked upon as suspicious or even rejected. However, "natural experiments" such as traumatic lesions, hemorrhage, and tumors provided by human cerebral pathology also destroy cell bodies and axons. That is why experimental neurophysiology was so triumphant before 1983: it could reproduce and explain the comas and insomnia of human neurology. The association of a lesion of cell bodies and axons may often be of great topographical diagnostic value, but it does not always help assess function. This is the basic problem of localizationists and non-localizationists.

New actors have appeared on the cerebral stage. We are beginning to glimpse the major role of glia in cortical energy processing. The brain is a machine that consumes a lot of energy as glucose. It is likewise a machine that both commands and depends on the whole organism. Two experiments, among many others, have helped us understand the complexity of this form of regulation.

The so-called neutral temperature for most mammals is 27°C (at 27°C the organism, and therefore the brain, does not utilize energy as a defense against cold or heat). Progressive body hypothermia from 37°C to 27°C can be achieved by suppression of central mechanisms of defense against cold. This can sometimes trigger a cascade of surprising events. The duration of paradoxical sleep increases. It releases paradoxical mechanisms of heat loss by vasodilation. Body temperature thus decreases. Thus, through "illogical" positive feedback mechanisms, a loop is set up to conserve energy by lowering temperature and, therefore, glucose consumption. Periods of paradoxical sleep get longer and longer, and each contributes to the lowering of body temperature, so that at 25 °C paradoxical sleep is continuous. We mentioned the $Q_{10}$ law in chapter 1, according to which a decrease of 10 °C in body temperature halves most biological processes (metabolism, oxygen consumption, heart rate, respiration). We know that paradoxical sleep lowers brain temperature but we do not know why dreaming avoids the $Q_{10}$ law. At what stage is Nature permitted to laugh at biologists?

It is very obvious that all new knowledge contributes to the destruction of fundamental concepts on which it may have been based at the outset. This is why, like the ruination and dismantling of the empires of Eastern Europe, the development of neuroscience has left a trail of ruins of fundamental concepts on which the neurophysiology of the sleep-wake cycle was established.

Between 1950 and 1980 it was accepted "classically" that the midbrain reticular formation and parts of the hypothalamus were responsible for arousal (see chapter 2). Their destruction, either by trauma in humans or electrolytic lesion in animals, was consistently followed by prolonged coma. But the destruction of only the cell bodies in these nuclei did not disturb waking. The coma was therefore due to the interruption of various ascending and descending pathways coming from the lower brainstem or from the cortex. We now know of numerous redundant and interconnected systems that maintain waking. It could hardly be otherwise, for tens ôf millions of years of evolution have contributed to the perfection of redundant mechanisms and circuits for maintaining the waking state that is indispensable to the survival of the individual and the species.

For a long time, recording of electrical activity of neurons constituted the alpha and omega of our knowledge of the brain. If a given group of neurons was active during waking and inactive during sleeping or dreaming, one might deduce that these neurons were responsible for waking, or certain phenomena related to waking. It is not certain that such reasoning is correct. Some groups of neurons could very well be active during waking in order to induce a cascade of processes leading to sleep and dreams.

So the neurophysiologist can no longer entirely trust electrophysiology. He must try to deduce the diachronic relationship (which might last some minutes, or even an hour) between the release of a neurotransmitter (such as serotonin) and the different intracellular postsynaptic messages which trigger a feedback loop leading to sleep, and thus the ceasing of activity in a system.

These few examples have contributed to the overthrow of certain concepts of causality on which the neurophysiology of the 1960s was based. The ever-increasing complexity of our view of brain organization has rendered obsolete the concept of necessary and adequate conditions for the appearance of a state of vigilance. This concept had managed to establish a role for the reticular formation in arousal because a lesion in it caused coma and its stimulation caused arousal. It is no longer valid in view of the intricacy of the innumerable neuronal and glial systems responsible for sleep-wake cycles. This is why we tend more and more to admit that it is an ensemble of conditions adequate for the appearance of dreams that really causes dreams.

We still have not found a "sleep molecule" that can send a patient with insomnia to sleep physiologically. But there is an ever-growing list of sleep "factors" that increase sleep in a rat by 10% or 20%. At the moment, most attention is being given to adenosine and $\gamma$-aminobutric acid (GABA). GABA is a favored candidate for a physiological "sleeping pill" if we can find the strategic point at which it acts and which receptors it affects.

Advances in the field of biological clocks have not upset physiologists who study cats, because our favorite animal, unlike Lewis Carroll's rabbit, rarely looks at his watch before going to sleep, for he does not have a circadian rhythm for sleeping. Melatonin made a tumultuous entry onto the stage of sleep. We saw in chapter 1 that it is the hormone of the pineal gland, implicated in circadian rhythms. We first thought it might be *the* veritable hypnogenic factor, as well as being the hormone of youth and health. It is a "chronobiological" substance, that has proved of great interest in treating disturbances of the human sleep clock, such as jet lag and certain other forms of sleep disturbance. But, in spite of the enormous media attention it has attracted, it is not the "sleep hormone."

Societies for the study of sleep have multiplied in both thematic and geographical terms. The evolution of sleep research in the last decade has been marked by a relative decrease in interest in fundamental problems and more emphasis on clinical applications. The domain of sleep research has been invaded by "sleep medicine." Sleep medicine and sleep clinics have taken giant steps forward, especially in the United States.[93] For example, sleep apnea, which we mentioned in chapter 1, has become a medical specialty, and a mixed bag of respiratory physicians, ear-nose-and-throat specialists, and neurologists attend symposia devoted to sleep pathology. Studies of snoring (apnea during sleep) and impotence (whether you have erections during your dreams) have become highly lucrative specialties. In short, our world has changed. Epidemiological studies, again mainly in the United States, have made us aware of the considerable cost of disturbances of daytime alertness, especially related to various kinds of accident, such as those involving automobiles and the workplace. Daytime dozing has become a greater menace than insomnia. Europe has followed the trend, but with a certain delay!

Basic science researchers, looking for the mechanisms and functions of sleeping and dreaming, are less numerous. It needs many years to acquire expertise in physiology, biochemistry, pharmacology, and anatomy in order to be able to penetrate the mysteries of the sleeping brain. Unfortunately, there are not many old professors left capable of teaching the integrated physiology of waking and sleeping. Grant proposals are now less likely to be successful, and many departments of physiology have had to change their name to be more acceptable. My old Laboratory for the Neurobiology of Vigilance was rebaptized the Laboratory of Molecular Oneirology.

## A Physiological Advance: The Erection of Dreaming

Some physiological discoveries about sleep have opened new horizons. We can accept that the problem of the conscious content of dreams is related to the cognitive *sub*conscious. I might cite some discoveries related to the "affective" subconscious. I believe that there has been a revolution in this respect in the last decade. In particular there is the question of erection during dreaming or, to be more objective, during paradoxical sleep. Here we are confronted by numerous mysteries.

The first mystery is that erection accompanies every period of paradoxical sleep, whether it contains erotic scenes or not, and independent of the dreamer's age, from birth to old age. Although erection is easy enough to see in a subject lying on his

back, it was not described scientifically until 1944,[117] and more
fully in 1965.[47] So, Why was this? In fact it was observed a
long time ago. In the famous well scene in the Lascaux cave,
painted 18,000 years ago by our Cro-Magnon ancestors, we
see a sleeping man with his arms outstretched, apparently
sleeping soundly, and with a full erection (see cover illustra-
tion). A bird is perched beside him. In front of him are a
wounded bison, with its entrails hanging out, and a broken
spear. According to some prehistorians this is a scene related
to shamanism. But I can think of another interpretation. The
association of erection in a prostrate figure with a bird might
provide a clue to the interpretation of his cave painting. I
assume that our ancestors were capable of observation and that
they had already noticed periods of erection during the night,
in infants as in old men. Maybe they had related these intui-
tively to dreaming. So how did they interpret dreams? Probably
in a similar way as at the dawn of all civilizations, as we discussed at the beginning of chapter 2. How could they interpret
the illogical, magical dream images of flying or levitation without recourse to concepts of spirit or soul? These immaterial
elements leave the inert, material body and fly away like a bird
to wander through space and time. So we visit the past through
dreams of our previous experiences, or the future through
premonitory dreams. The artists of Lascaux dreamed of their
desire to kill a bison.

You may think this a wild and presumptuous hypothesis.
Maybe. But I have just discovered in a book on Napoleon's
expedition to Egypt a drawing of a bas-relief from the walls of
the Great Temple of Denderah, from the Third Dynasty (figure
21). It pictures a reclining man with an obvious erection. The
ba, the spirit or soul of the Egyptians, is again represented

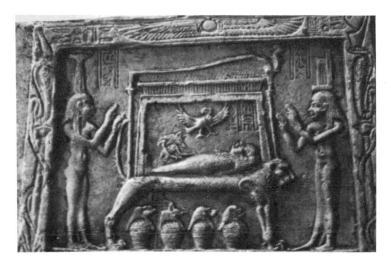

**Figure 21**
Bas-relief from the walls of the Great Temple of Denderah (Third Dynasty).

by a bird with a human head. An erection and a bird: again, perhaps a dream.

Now we have to find a nonmetaphysical explanation for erection during dreaming. Erection is part of sexuality, and therefore of affect. It is a peripheral expression of the affective unconscious, for we cannot suppress the erection of dreaming voluntarily. How could such an obvious sign, described 18,000 years ago, be forgotten by science, even hidden, until 1944? Later Charles Fisher further described and recorded erection during dreaming, even in the absence of erotic overtones.[47] It is true that Fisher, apart from being a great physiologist, had been a Freudian psychoanalyst for some years. I have no valid explanation for the disappearance of interest in dream erection for thousands of years. Certainly, the three great monotheistic religions tended to censor the phenomenon. Dreams were divine messages to dreamers, but if they were accompanied by an erection it might suggest some influence from the devil! Of course, the rediscovery of erection during dreaming delighted the disciples of Freud. This proved for them that all dreams had a sexual connotation, and that they were right to look for the explanation of dreams in their "latent" content: a pipe in a dream had nothing to do with smoking, but was a phallus.

This proof of sexual monism in dreams was a comfort to certain schools of psychoanalysis which interpreted dreams according to a sexual monism dear to Freud himself, and helped give a modicum of physiological credibility to psychoanalysis in the 1960s and 1970s. Neurobiologists remained silent, for they had no experimental physiological arguments to be able to counterattack. The male was put on a pedestal, but he was soon followed by the female, who enjoys the same phenomenon, but only recordable with difficulty. The human was different from the other animals, which do not have erections during paradoxical sleep, or so one thought. The affective, sexual subconscious was a characteristic of the human brain: it alone contained the machinery of desire.

The discovery of erection in the *rat* during paradoxical sleep knocked man off his sexual pedestal on the one hand, and on the other hand opened the possibility of using the rat's oneiric erection to guide us, like Ariadne's thread, through the labyrinth of dreaming. "Life is short, research long and difficult," to paraphrase Hippocrates. In 1992 a young researcher from the University of Ohio, Markus Schmidt, came to spend four years in my laboratory. He was very interested in the mechanisms of erection, so I suggested that he look for erection during sleep in the rat. Even if people thought it did not exist, I told him that absence of proof is not proof of absence. We had available the necessary instruments in the form of microcatheters, and Markus was very skillful. After a number of failures, which is par for the course in research, we soon became convinced that erection did exist in rats during paradoxical sleep.[143] It was not a constant feature, only occurring about half the time. So, should we lower man to the level of the rat, or place the rat on the same pedestal as man? Neurobiologists could now reply to the Freudians. Dream erection existed in rats, and probably in most mammals. The trigger centers were located in the hypothalamus. We traced the descending pathways. Now we can tackle the problem of why an erection takes place, as long, that is, as there are still enough interested researchers.

Why does erection accompany some, but not all, periods of paradoxical sleep in rats? Is there a programming mechanism that sometimes selects an erection, but not always? This would imply organization in time and in space. I sometimes dream myself of a Laboratory of Experimental Psychoanalysis to follow in the footsteps of the Laboratory for Molecular Oneirology, where we would study electrical activity during erection in paradoxical sleep in virgin, prepubertal rats, or others exposed to sexually active females.

### The Role of Molecular Biology in Sleep Research

A new generation of researchers, young and enthusiastic, masters of the tools of molecular biology, has invaded our laboratories.[83] They compensate for their ignorance of the old sleep literature (more than three years old, that is) by their great temerity in their search for the gene or genes responsible for sleeping and dreaming. This is a treasure hunt replete with jargon that only the initiated understand.

As we have already seen, molecular biology has pervaded sleep research at several levels. In the field of molecular genetics, the genes responsible for human and canine narcolepsy[115] have been isolated. But I do not believe that gene therapy of narcolepsy is for tomorrow.

Molecular genetics is replacing classical genetics. In some approaches pure chance plays a capital role. I am thinking especially of experiments using "knockout" mice, in which a gene that is suspected of being of interest in suppressed (or "knocked out"). Almost every month, as in the Comedia della Arte, a new diva appears, a knockout mouse with a key gene removed. Of several dozen strains examined so far, none have produced spectacular results, apart from 10% or 20% variations in the amount of sleep.

It has become fashionable to explore putative differences in gene expression between waking and sleeping animals using very precise methods. I wish researchers pursuing this route the best of luck. The young genetic engineers will learn, as older neurophysiologists discovered when they observed recovery of sleep after brain lesions, that the ablation of a gene, like a brain lesion, can be compensated by other systems. Redundancy is the keyword in systems that have been around for tens of millions of years.

The development of techniques to visualize "immediate early" genes (such as *c-fos*) has given us some encouraging results, without, however, opening up a terra incognita. These techniques have enabled verification of the detailed topography of brain areas implicated in the triggering of slow wave or paradoxical sleep. We are able to almost double the duration of paradoxical sleep in cats by blocking a part of the brainstem that normally inhibits paradoxical sleep,[138] but we wanted to know the topography of any higher centers involved. So we identified regions where there was a correlation between the number of neurons expressing the *c-fos* gene that had been excited during paradoxical sleep and the duration of this paradoxical sleep. We found the most significant correlation in the hippocampus and the amygdala.[140] Could these two structures be implicated in the process of the programming of individuality?

## Images of the Living Brain

Certain recent findings in man using PET scanning also draw attention to limbic structures activated during paradoxical sleep.[105] An extension of this approach seems promising, an approach that enables us to see the function of the brain in three dimensions during the sleep-wake cycle. So the majority of researchers are waiting with bated breath for the results of studies combining PET scanning, "functional" magnetic resonance imagines (fMRI), magnetoelectroencephalography, and tomographic electroencephalography. When these methods become faster, physiologists' dreams may become reality: to see the brain working in real time, during waking, during sleep, during dreams, daydreams, and even lucid dreams. At the same time, just as the spectroscope enabled us to penetrate the inner secrets of the stars, our own dream of being able to penetrate the energy mechanisms of the brain with spectroscopic magnetic resonance, seems to be getting closer.

Results of PET scanning during waking mental tasks are already very interesting. For example, if you ask a sportsman to imagine that he is taking part in a race, you see that the motor areas of the cerebral cortex are very active although there is no muscle activity. There can also be increased heart rate and breathing just as if the subject was in the race.[30] So mental images, such as those in the sportsman, are good examples of acquired or epigenetic programming enabling enhanced motor performance. Perhaps during paradoxical sleep similar mechanisms to those revealed by PET scanning during mental images could be controlled by the hippocampus or the amygdala and could play a similar role by facilitating certain neuronal circuits.

**The Ecological Approach**

In 1998 I visited the French Crozet and Kerguelen Islands in the southern Indian Ocean. I was particularly interested in the day and night life in the colonies of 50,000 king penguins. They must constantly defend their minute territory of about one square meter from their neighbors with their beaks and wings, up to 5000 times a day! They thus have no time for sleep, which is, however, easy to observe in isolated penguins. They spend periods of several weeks when they get little or no sleep. We are only at the beginning of studying sleep in "ecological" conditions, made possible by miniaturized electronic transmitters, that will certainly furnish much more interesting results than laboratory studies. So sleep research is going to need a lot more time and patience.

**The Ultimate Problem: The Function of Dreams**

Physiology is the study of function, the study of the mechanisms of basic processes with obvious functional goals—circulation, respiration, nutrition, reproduction, salt and water balance, vision, visuomotor coordination, memory, learning, and many others. It is easy to study such processes to check that the function is properly catered for. The physiologist can vary the inputs to a system to understand the different regulatory mechanisms that are involved. For example, after water deprivation, what intra- or extracranial receptors are sensitive to osmolarity, what signals do they emit, and how and where do hormonal regulatory systems act? But the neurophysiologist who studies dreams can offer neither cause nor function. He cannot order up paradoxical sleep and can only note the presence of an apparently spontaneous brainstem pacemaker. The only variables at his disposal are strange quantities and irrational numbers, such as the amount and duration of paradoxical sleep. Respiratory rate signifies something for the organism that the physiologist can appreciate. The duration of a dream does not.

So, the hypno-oneirologist has a very strange stature in neuroscience. He knows that there is no obvious real cause for sleep and dreams, but rather a constellation of adequate conditions that must all be present. Generally, the last experimental condition is held to be causal. But this researcher is still searching for a cause, and so remains divorced from function.

We must then admit our considerable ignorance when we study sleep or dreams. Even if our intuition tells us that one of the roles of sleep is to save brain energy, we also know that it serves to prepare adequate conditions for the appearance of dreams. But why has evolution built a brain that, while asleep, is periodically subject to a mechanism that delivers fantastic images, paralyzes our muscles, suppresses our homeostatic systems, and gives us an erection? We know a lot of "how" without knowing "why," because we are not capable of detecting changes in behavior, in the brain or in the organism, when we suppress paradoxical sleep or dreams in animals or man.

It is obvious that the understanding of the logic of sleeping and dreaming depends on finding the appropriate level. It does not seem that the sleeping or dreaming brain will be explained by putting together our knowledge about all the molecules involved, or of a genetic program. Complexity has its own laws.

Has our generation been blind since 1960? The next generation will be astonished at our blindness, not realizing that it, too, is blind to its own blindness.

# Glossary

**Acetylcholine**  One of the neurotransmitters, released at certain synapses to propagate a nerve impulse to the next neuron, or to a muscle.

**Aerobic**  A type of metabolism using oxygen, used by most animal tissues under normal conditions. It is described by the Krebs cycle.

**Amygdala**  A nucleus of the brain deep within the temporal lobe, associated with affective behavior.

**Anaerobic**  A type of metabolism without oxygen, used by certain organisms or tissues and which produces lactate as a byproduct.

**Atonia**  Lack of muscular contraction, resulting in virtual paralysis, as during paradoxical sleep.

**ATP**  (adenosine triphosphate)  An important molecule in energy metabolism.

**Axon**  The single nerve fiber from the cell body of a neuron that conducts nerve impulses toward other neurons. Terminates at a synapse.

**Brainstem**  The part of the brain between the spinal cord and the thalamus. Consists of the medulla, pons, and midbrain.

**Catecholamines**  Chemical substances of the monoamine group, some of which are neurotransmitters (such as norepinephrine and dopamine)

**Chromosome**  Stringlike structures in cell nuclei that bear the genes.

**Circadian rhythm**  A biological rhythm of about one day. Cf. Ultradian rhythm

**Diachronic**  Evolving over a period of time.

**DNA (deoxyribonucleic acid)**    The molecular basis of the genes on the chromosomes of the cell nucleus.

**Dopamine**    A catecholamine neurotransmitter

**Epigenetic**    Processes, such as environmental ones, not strictly determined by genes.

**Epimethean evolution**    Epimetheus was the unpredictable brother of Prometheus. Natural selection is Epimethean in that it cannot predict, and only certain mutations can survive variations in the environment. Promethean evolution could anticipate future events.

**Genome**    Ensemble of genes that determine the hereditary characters in an individual.

**Glia**    Support cells of the central nervous system, distinct from the neurons (nerve cells). Take part in defense and nutrition of neurons.

**Glucose**    The form in which various sugars are used by the body for energy metabolism.

**Glycogen**    The common form in which glucose is stored in body cells to provide energy reserves.

**Hypnagogic images**    Images that appear when falling asleep.

**Hypnapompic images**    Images that appear when waking.

**Hypothalamus**    A region of the brain composed of numerous nuclei. Plays an important role in vital functions such as thirst, hunger, sexual behavior, sleep, temperature regulation, memory, emotion, and hormonal regulation via the pituitary gland.

**Lactate**    Byproduct of anaerobic metabolism.

**Lobe**    The cerebral hemispheres of the brain are formed of four lobes (frontal, parietal, occipital, and temporal), each with different sensory and motor functions.

**Medulla**    Part of the brainstem.

**Midbrain**    Part of the brainstem.

**Monoamines**    A group of chemicals, including the catecholamines (norepinephrine, dopamine) and serotonin, many of which are neurotransmitters.

**Neurotransmitter**    A chemical "messenger" that conveys nerve impulses across a synapse.

**Norepinephrine**    A monoamine neurotransmitter.

**Nucleus** 1. The central part of most cells containing the chromosomes that bear the genes. 2. An anatomically defined group of neurons.

**Ontogenesis** The development of an individual of a given species from the embryo.

**Paradoxical sleep** A state of the brain different from sleeping and waking, characterized by rapid eye movement (REM) and generalized muscular atonia. It coincides with periods of dreaming.

**Peptide** Chemical made of a short chain of amino acids. Has important functions in the central nervous system.

**PGO activity** Electrical brain activity closely associated with paradoxical sleep, responsible for rapid eye movements. Named because it is derived from the *pons*, and affects the lateral *geniculate* nucleus and *occipital* cortex of the visual system.

**Phenothiazine** A powerful "neuroleptic" chemical used to treat certain psychiatric conditions.

**Phylogenesis** The development of the species through evolution.

**Pineal gland** Gland attached to the brain near the brainstem. Takes part in circadian rhythms of sleep determined by light.

**Pituitary gland** Gland at the base of the brain secreting numerous important hormones. Attached to and controlled by the hypothalamus.

**Pons** Part of the brainstem.

**Promethean evolution** see Epimethean evolution.

**Reticular formation** Rather diffuse groups of neuronal nuclei in the brainstem, important in arousal.

**Serotonin (5-hydroxytryptamine, or 5-HT)** Monoamine neurotransmitter.

**Stochastic** Periodic repeats of a phenomenon in a random way.

**Synchronic** Happening at the same time.

**Synapse** The junction between the terminal of an axon and the next neuron or muscle.

**Ultradian rhythm** a biological rhythm that occurs several times a day. Cf. Circadian rhythm.

# Lexicon

The reader may sometimes be confused by the multiplicity of terms employed by different schools of physiology to designate the same phenomenon. This very multiplicity is proof that we still do not understand the mechanisms of sleeping and dreaming. For me, the most unfortunate term is that of *rapid eye movement (REM) sleep*. Does it apply to an eyeless mole, or to an owl that does not move its eyes?

Here is a nonexhaustive list of synonyms used to characterize sleeping and dreaming up to 1960.

## Sleep

Non-REM sleep

Orthodox sleep

Quiet sleep (during ontogenesis)

Slow wave sleep, containing two stages in the cat, and four in man.
  Stages 1 and 2, light sleep; 3 and 4, deep sleep

Synchronized sleep

Telencephalic sleep

## Dreaming

Activated sleep

Active sleep (during ontogenesis)

D state

Desynchronized sleep

Dreaming state
Emergent stage 1
Fast sleep
Paradoxical phase of sleep
Paradoxical sleep
REM sleep
Rhombencephalic phase of sleep
Stage 1 REM sleep

# References

1. Adrien J (1976). Lesion of the anterior raphe nuclei in the newborn kitten and the effects on sleep. Brain Research *103*:579–583.

2. Adrien J (1984). Ontogenèse du sommeil chez le mammifère. In: Physiologie du Sommeil. O Benoit (ed). Paris: Masson, pp 19–29.

3. Adrien J, Roffwarg HP (1974). The development of unit activity in the lateral geniculate nucleus of the kitten. Experimental Neurology *43*:261–275.

4. Aguilar-Roblero R, Arankowsky G, Drucker-Colin R, Morrison AR, Bayon A (1984). Reversal of rapid eye movement sleep without atonia by chloramphenicol. Brain Research *305*:19–26.

5. Allison T, Cicchetti DV (1976). Sleep in mammals: ecological and constitutional correlates. Science *194*:732–734.

6. Aserinsky E, Kleitman N (1953). Regularly occurring periods of eye motility, and concomitant phenomena, during sleep. Science *118*:273–274.

7. Baker TL, McGinty DJ (1979). Sleep-waking patterns in hypoxic kittens. Developmental Psychobiology *12*:561–575.

8. Berlucchi G (1965). Callosal activity in unrestrained, unanaesthetized cats. Archives Italiennes de Biologie *103*:623–634.

9. Bert J (1975). Caractères génériques et caractères spécifiques de l'activité de pointes "ponto-géniculo-occipitales" (PGO) chez deux babouins, *Papio hamadryas* et *Papio papio*. Brain Research *88*:362–366.

10. Bloch V, Dubois-Hennevin E, Leconte P (1979). Sommeil et mémoire. La Recherche *10*:1182–1191.

11. Bobillier P, Froment JL, Seguin S, Jouvet M (1973). Effets de la P-chlorophénylalanine et du 5-hydroxytryptophane sur le sommeil et le métabolisme central des monoamines et des protéines chez le chat. Biochemical Pharmacology 22:3077–3090.

12. Borbély AA, Tobler I (1989). Endogenous sleep-promoting substances and sleep regulation. Physiological Reviews 69:605–670.

13. Bosinelli M (1995). Mind and consciousness during sleep. Behavioral Brain Research 69:195–201.

14. Bouchard TJ (1984). Twins reared together and apart: what they tell us about human diversity. In: Proceedings of the Liberty Fund Conference on Chemical and Biological Bases for Individuality and Determinism. SW Fox (ed). New York: Plenum Press, pp 147–184.

15. Bouchard TJ, Lykken DT, McGue M, Segal NL, Tellegen A (1990). Sources of human psychological differences: the Minnesota study of twins reared apart. Science 250:223–228.

16. Bourguignon A (1968). Neurophysiologie du rêve et théorie psychanalytique. La Psychiatrie de l'Enfant 11:1–69.

17. Bovet D, Bovet-Nitti F, Oliverio A (1969). Genetic aspects of learning and memory in mice. Science 163:139–149.

18. Caillois R, von Grunebaum GE (1967). Le rêve et les sociétés humaines. NRF, Gallimard.

19. Campbell JH, Zimmermann EG (1982). Automodulation of genes: a proposed mechanism for persisting effects of drugs and hormones in mammals. Neurobehavior Toxicology Teratology 4:435–439.

20. Cespuglio R, Laurent JP, Jouvet M (1975). Etude des relations entre l'activité ponto-géniculo-corticale (PGO) et la motricité oculaire chez le chat sous réserpine. Brain Research 83:319–335.

21. Cespuglio R, Musolino R, Debilly G, Jouvet M, Valatx JL (1975). Organisation différentes des mouvements oculaires rapides du sommeil paradoxal chez deux souches consanguines de souris. Comptes Rendus de l'Académie des Sciences 280:2681–2684.

22. Chase MH, Morales FR (1985). Postsynaptic modulation of spinal cord motoneuron membrane potential during sleep. In: Brain Mechanisms of Sleep (DJ McGinty, A Morrison, R Drucker-Colin, PL Parmaggiani (eds). New York: Raven Press.

23. Chastrette N, Cespuglio R (1985). Effets hypnogènes de la desacetyl-α-MSH et du CLIP (ACTH 18–39) chez le rat. Comptes Rendus de l'Académie des Sciences 301:527–530.

24. Chouvet G (1981). Structures d'occurence des activités phasiques du sommeil paradoxal chez l'animal et chez l'homme. Doctoral thesis, Faculty of Sciences, University Claude-Bernard, Lyon, France.

25. Chouvet G, Blois R, Debilly G, Jouvet M (1983). La structure d'occurrence des mouvements oculaires rapides du sommeil paradoxal est similaire chez les jumeaux homozygotes. Comptes Rendus de l'Académie des Sciences 296:1063–1068.

26. Corner MA (1977). Sleep and the beginnings of behavior in the animal kingdom. Studies of ultradian motility cycles in early life. Progress in Neurobiology 8:279–295.

27. Crick F, Mitchison G (1983). The function of dream sleep. Nature 304:111–114.

28. Cudworth R (1678/1995). The True Intellectual System of the Universe London-Thoemmes.

29. Debru C (1990). Neurophilosophie du Rêve. Paris: Hermann.

30. Decety J, Perani D, Jeannerod M, Bettinardi V, Tadary B, Woods R, Mazziotta JC, Fazio F (1994). Mapping motor representations with positron emission tomography. Nature 371:600–602.

31. Delage Y (1919). Le rêve. Etude psychologique, philosophique et littéraire. Paris: Presses Universitaires de France.

32. Dement W (1960). The effect of dream deprivation. Science 131: 1705–1707.

33. Dement W (1972). Sleep deprivation and the organization of behavioral states. In: Sleep and the Maturing Nervous System. C Clemente, D Purpura, F Mayer (eds). New York: Academic Press.

34. Dement W, Kleitman N (1957). Cyclic variations in EEG during sleep and their relation to eye movements, body motility, and dreaming. Electroencephalography and Clinical Neurophysiology 9:673–690.

35. Dement WC (1981). Dormir, Rêver. Paris: Seuil.

36. Descartes R. Oeuvres. F Alquié (ed). Paris: Garnier.

37. Dewan EM (1970). The programing (P) hypothesis for REM sleep. International Psychiatric Clinics 7:295–307.

38. Drucker-Colin RR, Zamora J, Bernal-Pedraza J, Sosa B (1979). Modification of REM sleep and associated phasic activities by protein synthesis inhibitors. Experimental Neurology 63:458–467.

39. Ellis H (1925). The World of Dreams. Boston: Houghton Mifflin.

40. Everson CA (1995). Functional consequences of sustained sleep deprivation in the rat. Behavioral Brain Research 69:43–54.

41. Exner S (1894). Entwurf zu einer physiologischen Erklärung der psychischen Erscheinungen. Vienna: Deuticke.

42. Farbman AI (1990). Olfactory neurogenesis: genetic or environmental controls? Trends in Neuroscience 13:362–365.

43. Feinberg I, March JD (1995). Observations on delta homeostasis, the one-stimulus model of NREM-REM alternation and the neurobiologic implications of experimental dream studies. Behavioral Brain Research 69:97–108.

44. Feldman S, Conforti N (1985). Involvement of the sensory cortex in adrenocortical responses following photic and acoustic stimulation in the rat. Neuroscience Letters 55:249–253.

45. Fischer-Perroudon C, Mouret J, Jouvet M (1974). Sur un cas d'agrypnie (4 mois sans sommeil) au cours d'une maladie de Morvan. Effet favorable du 5-hydroxytrytophane. Electroencephalography and Clinical Neurophysiology 36:1–18.

46. Fisher C (1978). Experimental and clinical approaches to the mind-body problem through recent research in sleep and dreaming. In: Psychopharmacology and Psychotherapy: Synthesis or Antithesis. N Rosenzweig, H Griscom (eds). New York: Human Sciences Press, pp 61–96.

47. Fisher C, Gross J, Zuch J (1965). Cycle of penile erection synchronous with dreaming (REM) sleep. Archives of General Psychiatry 12:29–45.

48. Foulkes D (1966). The Psychology of Sleep. New York: Scribner's.

49. Fox PT, Raichle ME, Mintun MA, Dence C (1988). Nonoxidative glucose consumption during focal physiologic neural activity. Science 241:462–464.

50. Franck G, Salmon E, Poirrier R, Sadzot B, Franco G (1987). Etude du métabolisme glucidique cérébral régional chez l'homme, au cours de l'éveil et du sommeil par tomographie à émission de positrons. Revue d'Electroencephalographie et de Neurophysiologie Clinique 17:71–77.

51. Freud S (1895/1966). Project for a scientific psychology. In: Standard Edition of the Psychological Words of Sigmund Freud, vol 1. J Strachey (trans-ed). London: Hogarth Press, pp 283–297.

52. Freud S (1900/1953). The Interpretation of Dreams. In: The Standard Edition of the Complete Psychological Works of Sigmund Freud, vol 4. Strachey J (trans-ed). London: Hogarth Press.

53. Gackenbach J, LaBerge S (1988). Conscious Minds, Sleeping Brain. Perspectives on Lucid Dreaming. New York: Plenum Press.

54. Gastaut H, Broughton R (1965). A clinical and polygraphic study of episodic phenomena during sleep. Recent Advances in Biological Psychiatry 7:197.

55. Gélineau JB (1880). De la narcolepsie. Gazette des Hôpitaux 53:626–628, 635–637.

56. Gibson GE, Shimada M (1980). Studies on the metabolic pathway of the acetyl group for acetylcholine synthesis. Biochemical Pharmacology 29:167–174.

57. Giuditta A (1984). The neurochemical approach to the study of sleep. In: Handbook of Neurochemistry, 2nd ed. A Lajtha (ed). New York: Plenum Press.

58. Greenberg R, Pearlman C (1974). Cutting the REM nerve: an approach to the adaptive role of REM sleep. Perspectives in Biology and Medicine 17:513–521.

59. Greenough WT (1976). Enduring brain effects of differential experience and training. In: Neural Mechanisms of Learning and Memory. MR Rosenzweig, EL Bennett (eds). Cambridge, MA: MIT Press, pp 255–278.

60. Griffin DR (1982) Animal Mind—Human Mind. Munich: Springer-Verlag.

61. Hamburger V (1970). Embryonic motility in vertebrates. In: The Neurosciences. Second Study Program. FO Schmitt (ed). New York: Rockefeller University Press, pp 141–151.

62. Hasler AD, Scholz AT (1983). Olfactory Imprinting and Homing in Salmon. Berlin: Springer-Verlag.

63. Henley K, Morrison A (1969). Release of organized behavior during desynchronized sleep in cats with pontine lesion. Psychophysiology 6:245.

64. Hennevin E, Leconte P (1971). La fonction du sommeil paradoxal. Faits et hypothèses. Année Psychologique *71*:489–519.

65. Hennevin E, Leconte P (1977). Étude des relations entre le sommeil paradoxal et les processus d'acquisition. Physiology and Behaviour *18*:307–319.

66. Hirsch J (1962). Individual differences in behavior and their genetic basis. In: Roots of behavior. EL Bliss (ed). New York: Harper.

67. Hobson JA, McCarley RW (1977). The brain as a dreamstate generator: an activation-synthesis hypothesis of the dream process. American Journal of Psychiatry *134*:1335–1348.

68. Holden C (1980). Identical twins reared apart. Science *207*:1323–1328.

69. Holder N, Clarke JDW (1988). Is there a correlation between continuous neurogenesis and directed axon regeneration in the vertebrate nervous system? Trends in Neuroscience *11*:94–99.

70. Hopfield JJ, Feinstein DI, Palmer RG (1983). "Unlearning" has a stabilizing effect in collective memories. Nature *304*:158–159.

71. Horn G, Rose SPR, Bateson PPG (1973). Experience and plasticity in the central nervous system. Science *181*:506–514.

72. Jacobs BL, McGinty DJ (1971). Amygdala unit activity during sleeping and waking. Experimental Neurology *33*:1–15.

73. Jacobson M (1970). Development, specification, and diversification of neuronal connections. In: The Neurosciences. Second Study Program. FO Schmitt (ed). New York: Rockefeller University Press, pp 116–129.

74. Jeannerod M (1983). Le Cerveau-Machine: Physiologie de la Volonté. Paris: Fayard.

75. Jouvet M (1962). Recherches sur les structures nerveuses et mechanismes responsables des différentes phases du sommeil physiologique. Archives Italiennes de Biologie *100*:125–206

76. Jouvet M (1965). Paradoxical sleep. A study of its nature and mechanisms. Progress in Brain Research *18*:20–57.

77. Jouvet M (1974). Le rêve. La Recherche *5*:515–527.

78. Jouvet M (1978). Does a genetic programming of the brain occur during paradoxical sleep? In: Cerebral Correlates of Conscious Experience. PA Buser, A Rougeul-Buser (eds). Amsterdam: Elsevier.

79. Jouvet M (1979). Le comportement onirique. Pour la Science 25:136–152.

80. Jouvet M (1980). Paradoxical sleep and the nature-nurture controversy. Progress in Brain Research 53:331–346.

81. Jouvet M (1983). Hypnogenic indolamine-dependent factors and paradoxical sleep rebound. In: Proceedings of the Sixth European Congress on Sleep Research, Zurich. Basel: Karger, pp 2–18.

82. Jouvet M (1986). Programmation génétique itérative et sommeil paradoxal. Confrontations psychiatriques 27:153–181.

83. Jouvet M (1997). Le cycle veille-sommeil. Apport de la génétique et de la biologie moléculaire. Archives de Physiologie et de Biochimie 105:226–232.

84. Jouvet M, Delorme JF (1965). Locus coeruleus et sommeil paradoxal. Comptes Rendus de l'Académie des Sciences 159:895–899.

85. Jouvet M, Michel F (1958). Recherches sur l'activité électrique cérébrale au cours du sommeil. Comptes Rendus des Séances de la Société de Biologie 152:1167–1170.

86. Jouvet M, Michel F, Courjon J (1959). Sur un stade d'activité électrique cérébrale rapide au cours du sommeil physiologique. Comptes Rendus des Séances de la Société de Biologie 153:1024–1028.

87. Jouvet-Mounier D, Astic L, Lacote D (1970). Ontogenesis of the states of sleep in rat, cat and guinea pig during the first postnatal month. Developmental Psychobiology 2:216–239.

88. Kahn D, Pace-Schott EF, Hobson JA (1997). Consciousness in waking and dreaming: the roles of neuronal oscillation and neuromodulation in determining similarities and differences. Neuroscience 78:13–38.

89. Karnovsky ML, Reich P, Anchors JM, Burrows BL (1983). Changes in brain glycogen during slow-wave sleep in the rat. Journal of Neurochemistry 41:1499–1501.

90. Kitahama K, Valatx JL (1980). Instrumental and pharmacological paradoxical sleep deprivation in mice: strain differences. Neuropharmacology 19:529–535.

91. Kitahama K, Valatx JL, Jouvet M (1981). Paradoxical sleep deprivation and performance of an active avoidance task: impairment of c57BR mice and no effect in c57BL/6 mice. Physiology and Behavior 27:41–50.

92. Konishi M, Emlen ST, Ricklefs RE, Wingfield JC (1989). Contributions of bird studies to biology. Science 246:465–472.

93. Kryger MH, Roth T, Dement WC (1989). Principles and Practice of Sleep Medicine. Philadelphia: WB Saunders.

94. LaBerge SP (1985). Lucid dreaming: the power of being awake and aware in your dreams. Los Angeles: JP Tarcher.

95. LaBerge SP, Nagel LE, Dement WC, Zarcone VP (1981). Evidence for lucid dreaming during REM sleep. Sleep Research 10:148–181.

96. Laurent JP, Cespuglio R, Jouvet M (1974). Delimitation des voies ascendantes de l'activité ponto-geniculo-occipitale chez le chat. Brain Research 65:29–32.

97. Lavie P (1996). The Enchanted World of Sleep. New Haven, CT: Yale University Press.

98. Lichtenberg GC. Deutsche National Literatur 141:47–89.

99. Llinás RR, Paré D (1991). Of dreaming and wakefulness. Neuroscience 44:521–535.

100. Llinás R, Ribary U (1992). Perception as an oneiric-like state modulated by the senses. In: Induced Rhythms in the Brain. E Basar, TH Bullock (eds). Boston: Birkhäuser, pp 113–126.

101. Lopez-Garcia C, Molowny A, Garcia-Verdugo JM, Ferrer I (1988). Delayed postnatal neurogenesis in the cerebral cortex of lizards. Developmental Brain Research 43:167–174.

102. Lucero MA (1970). Lengthening of REM sleep duration consecutive to learning in the rat. Brain Research 20:319–322.

103. Magoun HW, Rhines R (1946). Inhibitory mechanism in bulbar reticular formation. Journal of Neurophysiology 9:165–171.

104. Mancia M (1995). One possible function of sleep: to produce dreams. Behavioral Brain Research 69:203–206.

105. Maquet P, Peters JM, Aerts J, Delfiore G, Degueldre C, Luxen A, Franck G (1996). Functional neuroanatomy of human rapid-eye-movement sleep and dreaming. Nature 383:163–166.

106. Matsuzaki M (1969). Differential effects of sodium butyrate and physostigmine upon the activities of para-sleep in acute brain stem preparations. Brain Research 13:247–265.

107. Mayes A (1983). Sleep Mechanisms and Functions in Humans and Animals. An Evolutionary Perspective. New York: Van Nostrand Reinhold.

108. Mayr E (1958). Behavior and Systematics. In: Behavior and Evolution. A Roe, GG Simpson (eds). New Haven, CT: Yale University Press, pp 341–362.

109. McCarley RW, Hobson JA (1977). The neurobiological origins of psychoanalytic dream theory. American Journal of Psychiatry 134:1211–1221.

110. Meddis R (1983). The evolution of sleep. In: Sleep Mechanisms and Functions in humans and Animals. An Evolutionary Perspective. A Mayes (ed). New York: Van Nostrand Reinhold.

111. Milner TA, Aoki C, Sheu KF, Blass JP, Pickel VM (1987). Light microscopic immunocytochemical localization of pyruvate dehydrogenase complex in rat brain: topographical distribution and relation to cholinergic and catecholaminergic nuclei. Journal of Neuroscience 7:3171–3190.

112. Moruzzi G, Magoun HW (1949). Brain stem reticular formation and activation of the EEG. Electroencephalography and Clinical Neurophysiology 1:455–473.

113. Mukhametov LM (1984). Sleep in marine mammals. In: A Borbély, JL Valatx (eds). Sleep mechanisms. Experimental Brain Research (suppl 8) 227–238.

114. Mukhametov LM, Supin AY, Polyakova IG (1977). Interhemispheric asymmetry of the electroencephalographic sleep patterns in dolphins. Brain Research 134:581–584.

115. Nishino S, Reid MS, Dement WC, Mignot E (1994). Neuropharmacology and neurochemistry of canine narcolepsy. Sleep 17:S84–92.

116. Nordeen EJ, Nordeen KW (1990). Neurogenesis and sensitive periods in avian song learning, Trends in Neurosciences 13:31–36.

117. Ohlmeyer P, Brilmeyer H, Hüllstrung H (1944). Periodische Vorgänge im Schlaf. Plügers Archiv für die gesamte Physiologie 258:559–560.

118. Ohno S (1976). Promethean evolution as the biological basis of human freedom and equality. Perspectives in Biology and Medicine 19:527–532.

119. Oniani TN (1988). Neurobiology of Sleep-Wakefulness Cycle. Tbilissi: Metsniereba.

120. Oppenheim RW (1985). Naturally occuring cell death during neural development. Trends in Neurosciences 8:487–493.

121. Orem J, Barnes CD (1980). Physiology in Sleep. New York: Academic Press.

122. Paton JA, Nottebohm FN (1984). Neurons generated in the adult brain are recruited into functional circuits. Science 225:1046–1048.

123. Perec G (1973). La Boutique Obscure. Paris: Denoël/Gonthier.

124. Perret JL, Tapissier J, Jouvet M (1979). Insomnie et mémoire. A propos d'une observation de dégénérescence striato-nigral. Electroencephalograpy and Clinical Neurophysiology 47:499–502.

125. Petitjean F, Buda C, Janin M, David M, Jouvet M (1979). Effets du chloramphenicol sur le sommeil du chat. Comparaison avec le thioamphenicol, l'erythromycine et l'oxytetracycline. Psychopharmacology 66:147–153.

126. Pompeiano O (1970). Mechanism of sensorimotor integration during sleep. Progress in Physiological Psychology 3:1–179.

127. Ramirez G (1973). Synaptic plasma membrane protein synthesis: selective inhibition by chloramphenicol in vivo. Biochemical and Biophysical Research Communications 50:452–458

128. Ramm P, Frost BJ (1983). Regional metabolic activity in the rat brain during sleep-wake activity. Sleep 6:196–216.

129. Rampin C, Cespuglio R, Chastrette N, Jouvet M (1991). Immobilisation stress induces a paradoxical sleep rebound in rat. Neuroscience Letters 126:113–118.

130. Rechtschaffen A (1967). Dream reports and dream experiences. Experimental Neurology (suppl 4):4–15.

131. Rechtschaffen A, Bergmann BM (1995). Sleep deprivation in the rat by the disk-over-water method. Behavioral Brain Research 69:55–63.

132. Rechtschaffen A, Vogle G, Shaikun G (1963). Interrelatedness of mental activity during sleep. Archives of General Psychiatry 9:536–547.

133. Robert W (1886). Der Traum als Naturnotwendigkeit erklärt. Hamburg.

134. Roffwarg HP, Muzio JN, Dement WC (1966). Ontogenetic development of the human sleep-dream cycle. Science 152:604–619.

135. Rose S, Kamin LJ, Lewontin RC (1984). Not in Our Genes: Biology, Ideology and Human Nature. New York: Pantheon.

136. Sakai K (1980). Some anatomical and physiological properties of pontomesencephalic tegmental neurons with special reference to the PGO waves and postural atonia during paradoxical sleep in the cat. In: The Reticular Formation Revisited. IBRO Monograph Series, vol 6. M Brazier (ed). New York: Raven Press.

137. Sakai K (1985). Anatomical and physiological basis of paradoxical sleep. In: Brain Mechanisms of Sleep. R Drucker-Colin, DJ McGinty, A Morrison, L Parmeggiani (eds). New York: Raven Press. pp 111–137.

138. Sallanon M, Denoyer M, Kitahama K, Aubert C, Gay N, Jouvet M. (1989). Long-lasting insomnia induced by preoptic neuron lesions and its transient reversal by muscimol injection into the posterior hypothalamus in the cat. Neuroscience 32:669–683.

139. Sastre JP, Jouvet M (1979). Le comportement onirique du chat. Physiology and Behaviour 22:979–989.

140. Sastre JP, Buda C, Kitahama K, Jouvet M (1996). Importance of the ventrolateral region of the periaqueductal gray and adjacent tegmentum in the control of paradoxical sleep as studied by muscimol microinjections in the cat. Neuroscience 74:415–426.

141. Sastre JP, Buda C, Lin JS, Jouvet M (1998). C-fos striato-septo hippocampal targets of paradoxical sleep. Sleep 14:164A.

142. Schenck CH, Bundlie SR, Ettinger MG, Mahowald MW (1986). Chronic behavioral disorders of human REM sleep: a new category of parasomnia. Sleep 9:293–308.

143. Schmidt MH, Valatx JL, Schmidt HS, Wauquier A, Jouvet M (1994). Experimental evidence of penile erections during paradoxical sleep in the rat. NeuroReport 5:561–564

144. Smith C (1985). Sleep states and learning; a review of the animal literature. Neuroscience and Biobehavioral Reviews 9:157–168.

145. Smith C (1995). Sleep states and memory processes. Behavioral Brain Research 69:137–145.

146. Smith C, Kitahama K, Valatx JL, Jouvet M (1974). Increased paradoxical sleep in mice during acquisition of a shock avoidance task. Brain Research 77:221–230.

147. Snyder F (1966). Toward an evolutionary theory of dreaming. American Journal of Psychiatry *123*:121–142.

148. Steriade M (1978). Cortical long-axoned cells and putative interneurons during the sleep-waking cycle. Behavioral and Brain Sciences *3*:465–483.

149. Steriade M, Hobson JA (1976). Neuronal activity during the sleep-waking cycle. Progress in Neurobiology *6*:1–376.

150. Steriade M, McCarley RW (1990). Brainstem Control of Wakefulness and Sleep. New York: Plenum Press.

151. Steriade M, Amzica F, Contreras D (1996). Synchronization of fast (30–40Hz) spontaneous cortical rhythms during brain activation. Journal of Neuroscience *16*:392–417.

152. Valatx JL, Jouvet D, Jouvet M (1964). Evolution électro-encéphalographique des différents états de sommeil chez le chaton. Electroencephalography and Clinical Neurophysiology *17*:218–233.

153. Vogel GW (1975). A review of REM sleep deprivation. Archives of General Psychiatry *32*:749–761.

154. Whyte LL (1960). The Unconscious before Freud. New York: Basic Books.

155. Wieland OH (1983). The mammalian pyruvate dehydrogenase complex: structure and regulation. Review of Physiology, Biochemistry and Pharmacology *96*:123–170.

156. Wiesel TN (1982). Postnatal development of the visual cortex and the influence of environment. Nature *299*:583–591.

157. Windle WF (1955). Regeneration in the central nervous system. Springfield, IL: Thomas.

158. Zhang JX, Valatx JL, Jouvet M (1987). Absence de rebond de sommeil paradoxal chez des rats hypophysectomisés et prétraités à la naissance par le glutamate de sodium. Comptes Rendus de l'Académie des Sciences *305*:605–608.

# Index

Note that page numbers followed by *f* indicate figures; those followed by *t* indicate tables.